Your Reiki Workout

Exercises and Meditations to
Explore the Wonder of Reiki

Build energy sensitivity, explore intent, develop your intuition,
create bespoke symbols, release blocked emotions

by Taggart King

www.reiki-evolution.co.uk
taggart@reiki-evolution.co.uk

978-1-9998852-2-9

About this book

This book started its life as a collection of downloadable 'self-help guides' that focused on particular issues that people needed help with:

- Getting started with Reiki
- Becoming more sensitive to the energy
- Developing your intuitive side
- Exploring the use of intent

What I have done in this book is to take these guides and re-write and expand upon them, so that you have here a practical workbook that you can use over time to explore the potentials that Reiki has to offer you.

But that is not all, because I have also included all the work that I have done in developing "Reiki synthesis", which is a way of using particular questions, and language forms, and a breathing technique to create bespoke symbols for yourself and others, and to deal with unhelpful emotions or beliefs.

Reiki synthesis focuses specific energies on freeing you from what is holding you back in your life, releases negative emotions and beliefs and creates specific energies to move you forward in the most powerful and positive way.

So this book is all about me making suggestions that you can follow to experiment for yourself, working on yourself and on other people, opening you up to your inner intuition and showing you how effortlessly you can control and direct the energies, sense the energies and develop your ability as a channel.

How to use this book

Don't read the whole book all in one go. It's not designed to be used like that. Take your time to work through the sections and exercises and actually carry out the exercises I am suggesting... don't just read about them and nod your head!

And take your time: this isn't a race. It's a journey where you develop your abilities and your sensitivities. You need to practise and reflect on how you are doing, try different things and see what happens.

Keep notes on your experiences as you go through the exercises and practices, and write down your thoughts and your questions so you can see how you progress over time.

Enjoy the journey.

I want you to scribble in this book!

This is a practical workbook, so I want to see you writing in it. Write in it anywhere: underline or circle things, put exclamation marks, arrows and asterisks, jot in the margins.

I hope that these ideas and exercises make a difference to you and that your practice of Reiki is enhanced as a result.

With best wishes,

Taggart King
Reiki Evolution
www.reiki-evolution.co.uk

Start with the basics

Get the basics right

The exercises detailed in this book have the potential to transform the way that you work with Reiki, but for them to be effective you first need to have a good basic routine of working with the energy.

So we start your adventures by you carrying out some simple energy exercises, which you should carry out every day, and which ideally you will continue with throughout these explorations and beyond.

To get the most out of this book and its exercises, you should really carry out these exercises for a couple of weeks before moving on to any of the other sections of this book.

Daily energy exercises

What you will find described below are energy exercises that you should carry out every day (or most days, in any case) and you can perform the exercises more than once a day if you like.

The exercises are designed to clear and cleanse your energy system, to get the energy flowing throughout your system, including your hands, and to focus the energy on your 'Tanden', an energy centre in your abdomen that is the centre of your personal universe.

These exercises were taught by Mikao Usui, according to a group of his surviving students, and were the first exercises his students embraced, so they are a good place to start!

If you are familiar with Japanese-style Reiki and are already practising "Hatsurei ho" regularly then the exercises below will be familiar to you (because you will already be using them!)

If you haven't heard of Hatsurei ho, these exercises will be new to you and I am sure you will enjoy them and get on very well with them.

Doing energy work on yourself, regularly, should be the foundation of your Reiki practice, no matter what lineage you trained in, and it's not really enough just to self-treat with Reiki if you want to get the most out of this book.

The energy exercises that I have for you produce the following effects.

They will:

1.   Clear and cleanse your energy system
2.   Help to move your energy system into balance
3.   Help to ground you
4.   Help to build up your personal energy reserves
5.   Develop your ability as a channel for Reiki
6.   Help to develop your sensitivity to the flow of energy
7.   Help to develop your intuitive side

The exercises focus on an area of your body called the "Tanden" ("Dantien" or "Tan T'ien" in Chinese) which is an energy centre located two fingerbreadths (3 – 5cm) below your tummy button and 1/3rd of the way into your body.

You will be imagining that you are drawing energy – or light – into the Tanden and then moving the energy on elsewhere.

The Tanden

The Tanden point is seen as the centre of our self from the Oriental point of view, a seat of power, the centre of our intuitive faculties, the centre of life. Drawing energy into your Tanden is drawing energy into the centre of your life and soul.

This area acts as a power centre that allows the amazing feats of martial artists to be performed, but also acts as the source of inspiration in Oriental flower arranging and calligraphy.

Meditation, exercise techniques like Tai Chi and QiGong, martial arts and Usui Reiki can all develop the Tanden, which is seen as your personal energy store, the focus of your personal power.

In energy cultivation techniques like Tai Chi and Qi Gong, the Tanden is the place where you store the energy that you are cultivating.

Conversely, martial artist might draw down energy from the sun to store in their Tanden before moving on to spar with an opponent.

The Tanden is also seen as the centre of your intuition and your creativity, so when people carry out Japanese calligraphy, or Ikebana (flower arranging) or the Tea ceremony, they are focusing their attention on the Tanden, the centre of their being.

Your Daily Energy Exercises

Mikao Usui taught his first degree students two simple exercises that they would carry out daily. The exercises are called "Kenyoku" and "Joshin Kokkyu Ho".

Kenyoku

This means 'Dry Bathing' or 'Brushing Off'.

Kenyoku can be seen as a way of getting rid of negative energy.

It has correspondences with Taoist massage, or meridian massage.

Here is what to do:

Stage 1: brushing down the torso

Place the fingertips of your right hand near the top of the left shoulder, where the collarbone meets the bulge of the shoulder.

The hand is lying flat on your chest.

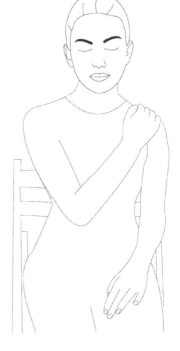

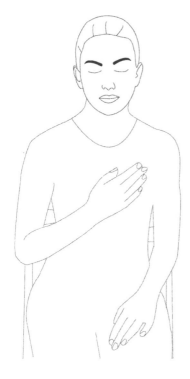

Draw your flat hand down and across the chest in a straight line, over the base of the sternum (where your breastbone stops and your abdomen starts, in the midline) and down to the right hip.

Exhale as you do this.

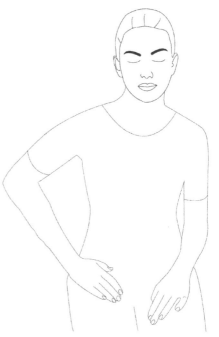

Do the same **on the right side**, using your left hand.

Draw your left hand from the right shoulder, in a straight line across the sternum, to the left hip, and again exhale as you make the downward movement.

Do the same **on the left side again** (like you did at the start), so you will have carried out movements with your right hand, left hand, and right hand again

Stage 2: brushing down the arms

Now put your right fingertips on the outer edge of the left shoulder, at the top of your slightly outstretched left arm, with your fingertips pointing sideways away from your body.

Move your right hand, flattened, along the outside of your arm, all the way to the fingertips and beyond, all the while keeping the left arm straight.

Exhale as you do this.

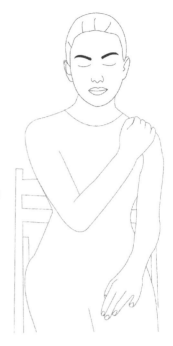

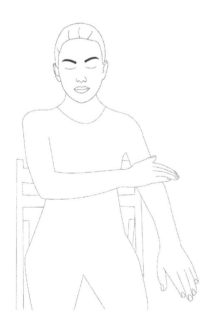

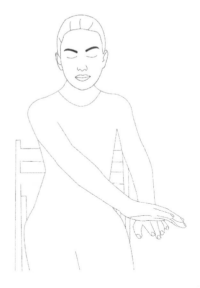

13

Repeat this process **on the right side**, with the left hand placed on the right shoulder, and move it down the right arm to the fingertips and beyond. Exhale as you do this.

Repeat the process **on the left side again**, so you will have carried out movements with your right hand, left hand, and right hand again, like before.

Why is this not symmetrical?

I realise that it may feel strange not to go, "right, left, right, left" and for some of you this can feel lop-sided and uneven, but all I can say is that this is how the exercise is carried out: with the order of right-left-right.

If you are right-handed, you could see this as giving emphasis to your 'dominant' hand.

If you really find that this sequence bothers you, you can experiment with making the movements symmetrical!

Joshin Kokkyu Ho

"Joshin Kokkyu ho" means 'Technique for Purification of the Spirit' or 'Soul Cleansing Breathing Method'.

This is a meditation that focuses on the Tanden point.

It is an exercise that clears and cleanses, grounds and balances, and it provides a powerful foundation for your energy work.

What to do

Put your hands on your lap with your palms facing upwards and breathe naturally through your nose

Focus on your Tanden point and relax.

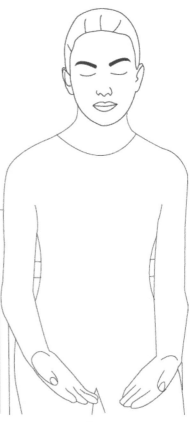

When you breathe in, visualise energy or light flooding into your crown chakra and passing into your Tanden, where it builds.

As you pause before exhaling, feel that energy expand throughout your body, melting all your tensions.

When you breathe out, imagine that the energy floods out of your body in all directions as far as infinity.

You should soon feel energy/tingling in your hands and even in your feet, as the meditation progresses!

It does not matter how you actually visualise the energy. Some people can visualise really easily, while others find it very difficult to 'see' a visual image in their mind's eye. This is not a problem because it is the underlying intent that is the important thing.

The energy moves in response to your intent.

For many people, visualising is a good way of focusing your intent in a particular way, but even with no imagined visual images, the energy will still move as you intend it to... so instead of visualising you might 'have in mind' or 'feel' or 'know' in some way that the energy is moving to a particular place, and that will work just as well.

So the energy will follow your thoughts, it follows your focus.

If you focus your attention or focus your awareness on your Tanden then you will be placing energy there, for example.

It is said that Ki is moved by the mind: "where the attention goes, ki flows"

Use this simple sequence

Follow these instructions to put together a short sequence of energy exercises*:

1. Close your eyes and take a few long deep breaths to calm yourself and to allow stress and tension to dissipate as you exhale
2. Focus your attention on your Tanden point
3. Perform Kenyoku
4. Perform Joshin Kokkyu Ho for 5-15 minutes
5. Be still for a while

If you are not used to meditating then you are likely to find that your mind wanders sometimes. This is normal and this is human, and you do not need to be perfect in order to achieve great benefits from using Reiki on yourself.

If thoughts intrude, pay them no attention; let them drift past and simply bring your attention back to what you were doing: focus your attention on your Tanden and again be open, and empty, feel yourself merging with the energy and becoming one with it, imagine yourself disappearing into the energy, and allow the energy to move in and out of you in time with your breath.

You observe any thoughts from a place of calm and stillness: you are not your thoughts. And with practice, over time, you should find that your mind will intrude less.

Note: (*) If you already know about and are practising "Hatsurei ho" then just keep on with this exercise daily, since it contains Kenyoku and Joshin Kokkyu ho, as you know.

Become more sensitive

People who learn Reiki come from all walks of life and react to the energy in different ways. Some people are more sensitive to the energy than others, even right from the start, and occasionally you might find someone attending a First Degree course, having done nothing with energy before, who is amazingly sensitive to the energy and is able to discern more than their Reiki teacher!

Most people will notice something happening when they work with energy on a First Degree course, whether working on themselves of treating other people, and the intensity of this experience will vary greatly from one person to another.

That's just the way it is.

But no matter how sensitive you are to the flow of energy to begin with, there are things that you can do to develop this sensitivity. The first thing that you can do is to work with energy regularly, for example treating yourself and also treating other people when you have the opportunity, and for many people this will help to increase the intensity of your experience of the flow of energy through you.

Unfortunately there is always a tendency to compare ourselves with other people, and if we come across another Reiki person who seems to be able to notice more in their hands than we do, or we read descriptions in a book or manual that talk about the things that some people have noticed when doing Reiki, we may feel inadequate or feel that we haven't been attuned properly or think that Reiki isn't working well for us.

Some of us may hold up an unattainable goal, telling ourselves that we can only do Reiki properly if we have a level of sensitivity that we do not have, and in fact do not need to have, and may not ever develop.

An interesting phenomenon I have observed is where a Reiki person will discount the sensations that they are experiencing in their hands and focus on the one, or two, sensations that they aren't currently experiencing.

So someone might complain that they don't feel heat in their hands, just fizzing and buzzing, and they feel inadequate as a result. At the same time, there will be another Reiki person somewhere who is dejected because all they can feel in their hands is intense heat, and not a hint of fizzing and buzzing!

Someone will complain that they can't really feel much in their hands: they just get a big light show in their mind's eye, while someone else thinks that their Reiki isn't working for them because all they get is physical sensations and no coloured lights at all!

Everyone is different and experiences the energy in different ways. There is no 'standard' way that people ought or should experience the energy. However you experience the energy is fine, and it doesn't matter what other people notice.

Interestingly, there are a few Reiki people out there who do not feel anything at all when they work on themselves and they do not feel anything when working on other people. I have met a few Reiki Masters who are in that category.

You might wonder what prompted them to continue their training, given that they had no experience of energy during First and Second Degree etc.

Well, they relied on and were encouraged and motivated by the positive responses that they were receiving from people that they practised on.

They could see that Reiki was doing something for the people that they were treating, even if they could not feel anything happening themselves, and they also focused on the positive changes that were happening within themselves since starting to work with Reiki.

They had all the evidence that they needed to show that Reiki was working for them.

That is why it is so important to work on yourself and to practice on other people: the more people you treat, the more positive feedback you are likely to receive about what you are doing, and that will encourage you.

If you feel that Reiki isn't working for you (because you can't feel too much going on in your hands) then you might decide not to treat people, where the feedback you could have received from the people you treated could have given you confidence in your ability.

You need to get out there and treat people!

Being very sensitive to the flow of Reiki within you, though, is not the be-all and end-all of your practice and we should not worry too much about the level of sensitivity that the universe has given us.

In fact, as we move on with our Reiki journey we tend to become more intuitive, and the development of an intuitive ability does make the issue of 'hand sensitivity' less important to us: if we can allow the energy to guide our hands to the right place to treat (for example using the 'Reiji ho' method') then we do not need to rely on 'scanning' to detect areas of need, and we can use intuition to guide us in terms of how long we might stay in a particular hand position, too.

We can carry out effective treatments by following a standard set of hand positions, of course, staying for longer in areas that seem to want to be treated for longer, and we can do this whether or not we can feel much happening in our hands.

So if you have two Reiki practitioners, one of whom is very, very sensitive to the energy and the other tends to feel very little going on in their hands, we should not conclude that the person who feels more is a better channel, or a more effective practitioner, or 'better attuned'; the issue of sensitivity to the energy is a personal thing and unrelated to that person's ability as a channel for the energy.

So, having been through all that, I want to tell you a little bit about this section of the book.

I have put this chapter together to provide you with some exercises that you can work with that should help you to develop your sensitivity to the energy over time.

There are no magic solutions, but If you persevere and work with the energy exercises that I suggest, and carry them out regularly, you should notice some positive changes.

Below you can read about different exercises you can try out and I suggest that you carry them out over several weeks.

You will need to find a few people to practice on if you are going to get the most out of this section. Some of the exercises you can carry out on your own, but not all of them.

What will I be doing?

1. Carrying out Kenyoku and Joshin Kokkyu ho every day: your baseline Reiki practice*
2. Learn a special meditation that you can use to bring energy into your hands
3. Learn to play with energy in different ways, on your own and with a partner

We have been teaching these methods on our live and home study courses for many years now, and these approaches seem to work for most people.

I wish you an exciting journey with this section of the book. Follow the instructions; get lots of practice (that's the key to it really), and you will be surprised by what is possible!

Have fun!

Note: (*) If you already know about and are practising "Hatsurei ho" then just keep on with this exercise daily, since it contains Kenyoku and Joshin Kokkyu ho, as you know.

Build energy in your hands

In this section I describe a special meditation you can carry out where you are drawing energy into and focusing your attention on your hands.

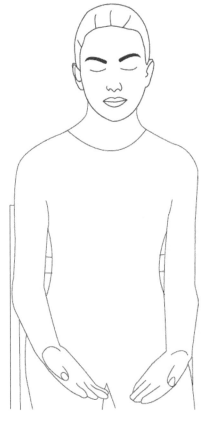

This meditation should be carried out in addition to the Kenyoku and Joshin Kokkyu ho (or Hatsurei ho) that you have been practising.

Carry out the 'hand energy meditation' each day; if you wish you can carry it out more than once a day.

Aim to carry out this exercise for a couple of weeks.

This is what to do

Put your hands on your lap with your palms facing upwards and breathe naturally through your nose.

Focus on your Tanden point and relax; still your mind.

When you breathe in, visualise energy or light flooding into your crown chakra and passing into your Tanden, building in your Tanden.

When you breathe out, imagine that the energy floods from your Tanden, along your arms, to your hands, where the energy then builds and becomes stronger and more intense in your hands.

With each out-breath you build up and intensify the energy in your hands.

The energy continues to build, to get stronger and heavier in your hands.

After a minute or two, start to become aware of your hands, how they feel. Focus your attention on your fingers, on the skin of your fingers, on your palms, on the skin of your palms.

- Can you feel any sort of sensation?
- Do they feel heavy or different in some way?
- Is there any throbbing or pulsing?
- Can you feel any fizzing or tingling?
- Is there warmth, or heat?
- Is there coolness or coldness?
- Is there some sort of a magnetic sensation?
- Do your hands feel different?

Continue with the exercise, breathing gently and normally, and moving energy in time with your breath, for several minutes.

Incidentally, it does not matter how you actually visualise the energy. Some people can visualise really easily, while others find it very difficult to 'see' a visual image in their mind's eye. This is not a problem because it is the underlying intent that is the important thing. The energy moves in response to your intent.

For many people, visualising is a good way of focusing your intent in a particular way, but even with no imagined visual images, the energy will still move as you intend it to… so instead of visualising you might 'have in mind' or 'feel' or 'know' in some way that the energy is moving to a particular place, and that will work just as well.

When you have completed the exercise, put your hands on yourself so the energy can dissipate into your body.

How does this feel?

Hand energy awareness exercise

Having spent some time building the energy in your hands using the meditation described above, you can now move on to another exercise where you practise becoming aware of energy sensations that are occurring naturally in your hands.

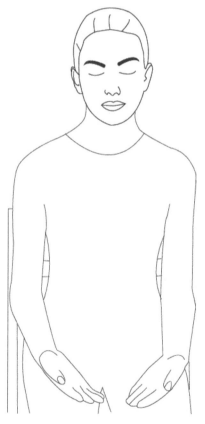

This is what to do

Put your hands on your lap with your palms facing upwards and breathe naturally through your nose.

Focus on your Tanden point and relax; still your mind.

After a minute or two, start to become aware of your hands, how they feel. Focus your attention on your palms, the heel of your palm, the centre of your palm, and where your palm meets your fingers.

Become aware of the skin covering your thumb and fingers, from the base to the tips. Focus your attention on your thumb and fingertips.

Then allow your attention to range across your palms and fingers, as is you were caressing the skin of your palm and fingers with your attention.

Be aware enough of what is happening in your hands to be able to answer these sorts of questions:

- What sort of sensations can you feel?
- Do you feel pressure or warmth?
- Do your hands feel heavy or different in some way?
- Is there any throbbing or pulsing?
- Is there heat or coolness?
- Is there a magnetic sensation?
- Can you feel any fizzing or tingling?
- In what way do your hands feel different?

Continue with the exercise for several minutes.

I spoke earlier about how Reiki will follow your focus and focus itself where your attention is directed. So just by focusing your attention on your hands, you are encouraging the energy to flood, settle and build there.

And free from any other distractions, your full attention is on your hands; this is a useful practice because you probably haven't spent much time considering the sensations in your hands in any sort of a focused or undistracted way.

You are helping your subconscious mind to understand what to do, giving it some practice in bringing to your attention sometimes subtle, often less-than-subtle, sensations as the energy builds and flows through your palms and fingers.

Use hypnotic suggestions

You might know that I trained as a Cognitive Hypnotherapist and NLP Master Practitioner with the Quest Institute at Regent's University and I have used my knowledge and experience of creating hypnotic suggestion patterns to create a series of Guided Reiki Meditations that combine the gentle power of Reiki with the potency of Ericksonian hypnosis.

Hypnotic suggestions can be very powerful on their own, of course, but I have discovered that when combined with Reiki they become particularly effective, as if the Reiki is in some way used as a 'carrier' to powerfully embed the suggestions in your subconscious mind.

Interestingly, Frank Arjava Petter, author of several books about Japanese style Reiki, and Hiroshi Doi, member of the Usui Reiki Ryoho Gakkai (Usui memorial society) describe a couple of techniques called Seiheki Chiryo and Nentatsu ho, both of which involve sending a thought or a positive affirmation into yourself or into a client, using Reiki as a way of helping to embed a useful idea or behaviour change.

Seiheki Chiryo means 'habit treatment technique' and Nentatsu Ho means 'send a thought technique'.

So using positive affirmations, or carefully-crafted suggestions, along with Reiki acting as some sort of a 'booster', has quite a good pedigree in the West and in the East!

I put together three collections of unique Reiki Guided Meditations which I tested extensively on a large group of Reiki volunteers they work fantastically well, and in fact they surpassed my expectations. It seems that when gentle suggestion patterns are combined with Reiki meditations, a very powerful combination is created, helping the listener to move powerfully in a new better direction.

The collection that you will probably be most interested in at the moment deals with Mindfulness, Energy Sensitivity and Developing Intuition.

I recommend that you listen to the 'energy sensitivity' track every day (the track lasts for about 12 minutes) for 4-6 weeks, during which time the beneficial changes develop and solidify.

One of my test subjects had to stop listening to the track after a couple of weeks because she found that she was becoming *too* sensitive!

So it's powerful stuff!

The Nentatsu Ho Meditations can be found on the Reiki Evolution web site for immediate download:

www.reiki-evolution.co.uk

Playing with energy

In this section you are going to start to 'play' with energy, on your own and with a partner, just to see what you might notice. Don't expect to feel a particular sensation, don't anticipate a particular level of intensity, keep an open mind and just mess around, and see what happens.

Have fun with it. You need to be light-hearted and playful. Do not worry about what you are feeling.

I have suggested five different exercises that you can carry out; do them often, and not just once or twice.

What you are doing is practising focusing your attention on, or tuning into, the energy in you, in your hands, and the energy around you and around other people.

I suggest that you carry out these exercises on people who have already been attuned to Reiki, if you can, because they are likely to be more sensitive to the energy and its movements and they will probably be able to give you more useful feedback than people who have not been attuned.

But these exercises will still be of benefit if you can only work with non-attuned people. Non-attuned people can sometimes be surprisingly sensitive to the energy!

I suggest that you carry out these exercises on a few different people, so you can feel the energy field of, and experience the flow of energy through your hands into, different subjects.

Carry out these exercises for a couple of weeks.

Energy Between your Hands

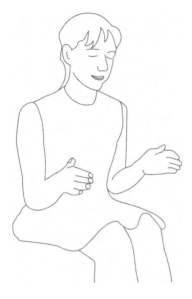

Rub your hands together for half a minute, rather like you are warming your hands up after being out in the cold.

Now hold your hands out in front of you, shoulder width apart, with your palms facing each other, rather like you were holding the sides of a very large ball.

Now slowly 'bounce' your hands together until you have an impression that there is something tangible between your hands.

You may feel something squashy like a marshmallow, a balloon or a rubber ball; you may feel a surface, a layer, some resistance, some magnetic repulsion… some 'thing' that your hands are resting on that prevents them from touching.

Now obviously you can move your hands all the way together if you want to, but with a few attempts most people can experience something between their hands that they can rest their hands on, bounce their hands against.

Sometimes you can find a position where your hands don't want to come any closer, but equally they don't want to move away from each other either: a position of balance.

You are experiencing your energy field.

You have always been able to do this. It has always been right there in front of you.

To experience it you have simply changed your focus.

Energy on a Partner's Hand

You will need someone to do this exercise with you. Sit fairly near to each other. Both of you should rub your hands together for half a minute, rather like you are warming your hands up after being out in the cold.

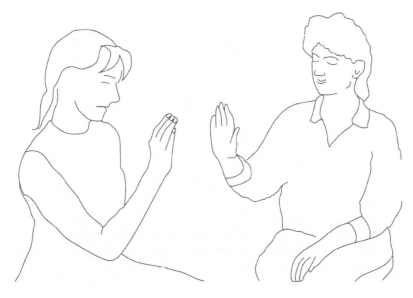

Now hold one hand out in front of you, at shoulder height, with your palm facing your partner's palm, rather like you were about to push his/her hand away from you or give a rather low 'high five'!

Now slowly 'bounce' your hands together until you have an impression that there is something tangible between your hands.

You may notice something squashy like a marshmallow, a balloon or a rubber ball; you may experience a surface, a layer, some resistance, some magnetic repulsion... some 'thing' that your hands are resting on that prevents them from touching.

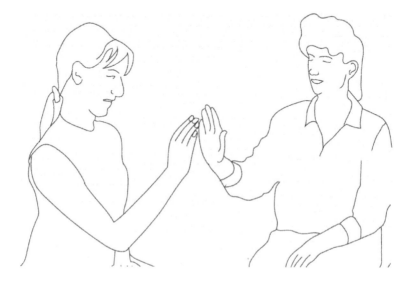

See if you can agree between yourselves about the point where you can both experience that 'contact', that layer or surface, that magnetic repulsion or resistance.

Now one person should keep their hand still while the other person slowly moves their hand vertically up and down, from side to side, and slowly towards and away from their partner's palm.

- How does this seem?
- What sensations are you experiencing?
- How does your experience change?

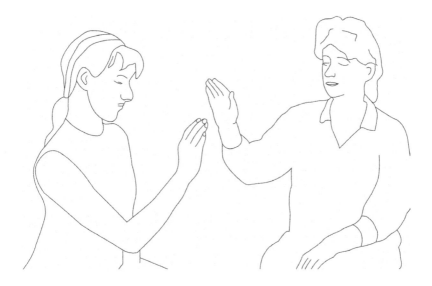

Now swap over: the person whose hand was moving should now keep their hand still, and the other person moves their hand around (as described above).

- Again, how does this seem?
- What sensations are you experiencing?
- How do the sensations change?
- What impressions do you have?

Now both move your hands, together and away from each other. Just go with the flow and see where they want to go.

You are experiencing the other person's energy field, and you are noticing the reaction of your energy field to the other person's energy field. You have always been able to do this. It has always been right there in front of you. To experience this you have simply changed your focus

Energy around Head & Shoulders

You will need someone to do this exercise with you.

One person sits in a dining chair and closes their eyes. They are the 'guinea pig' and just sit there throughout the exercise. The other person stands behind them.

The person standing up starts with their hands raised, hovering about 12" (30cm) above the subject's head, palms down.

Now bring your hands slowly down, bouncing them down until you feel or have the impression in some way that your hands are resting on the subject's energy field.

Now move your hands away again and 'bounce' them down onto an adjacent area above the head. Experience the energy field over different parts of the subject's head, the forehead, the back of the head and the temples.

- Is the energy field the same distance away all round the head?
- Does it seem the same in all places?
- If not, what are its qualities?
- How does the energy feel to you?

Experience the energy field over the shoulders, above, behind and in front.

- How does the energy field seem here?

Does the energy field feel bright, lively, fizzy or buzzy? Or does it seem dull in some way? Does it strike you as heavy and solid, or does it appear light and ethereal? Does the quality of the energy bring a particular thought or emotion?

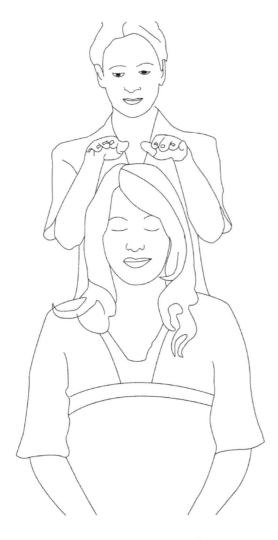

Push Someone off Balance

You will need someone to do this exercise with you.

Your 'victim' should stand up, standing still with their eyes closed. They should not stand stiff and rigid, but simply stand in a relaxed way, and they should be told that if they feel that their body wants to drift either forwards or backwards then they should not resist: they should simply allow their body to drift, and if they need to take a step back to steady themselves then they should do that.

Stand about 2m (6ft) behind the person with your hands in front of your chest, palms facing away from you and towards the victim, as if you were going to push their shoulders.

Slowly move towards them until you have an impression that your hands are resting on the person's energy field.

You may have some physical sensations – maybe the same or similar to the sensations you experienced when you were feeling the energy field in the above exercises – or you may simply 'know' that your hands have made contact with the person's energy field.

Now you are going to slowly alternate between doing two things:

Deliberately 'squash' the person's energy field for 20-30 seconds, moving your palms closer and closer to their body intending that you are compressing their energy field against them.

Deliberately pull their energy field away from their body
for 20-30 seconds, by moving your palms away from their
body. You can take a step back. You can take several steps
back, and you imagine that their energy field is being
stretched out like elastic, being pulled away from their body.

Do not alternate quickly between pushing and pulling. That
won't work.

You need to be either squashing their energy field for a while,
or pulling it away from their body for a while.

Alternate between the two.

What happens?

Most people will find that they lean forward or backwards.
People lean back more readily than they move forward.
Some people will resist and although you cannot see any
movements, they can feel the pull. Some people are pulled
backwards so powerfully that they have to take a step back
to steady themselves.

Your body is used to being in the centre of its energy field,
and if you distort that then your body seems to want to drift
into a position of balance.

Please note that if the person wants to resist this, they can.
The effect is subtle, but noticeable, and can always be
resisted. The exercise will only be successful if the guinea
pig is willing to allow their body to drift. Sometimes there can
be an 'ego thing', particularly with men, who do not want to
admit to feeling anything, and certainly do not want to show
any 'weakness' by being pushed by someone.

Play with 'Energy Balls'

You will need someone to do this exercise with you.

Hold your hands approximately 9" (22cm) apart and imagine that energy is flooding through your palms into the space between. Imagine that the energy ball is becoming stronger, denser, and more intense; you are building up a ball of energy between your hands.

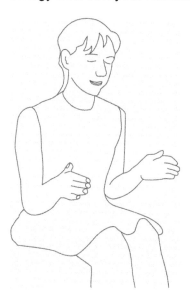

What can work well is to imagine that, with each gentle out-breath, you are flooding the space between your hands with energy; as you breathe in, imagine the energy building and getting stronger between your hands; as you breathe out again, flood more energy into the space between your hands.

You don't need to flood energy into the space between your hands on every out-breath; it can work very nicely to alternate your breaths in and out, with one in/out cycle being about flooding the energy, and the next cycle being about allowing that energy to build and intensify.

Bounce your hands against this ball of energy and feel it become stronger and denser over a period of several minutes.

You might feel that you want to 'compact' the ball of energy on the out-breath, making it more dense and strong, while on the in-breath you allow your hands to drift apart to an extent. Do whatever feels most appropriate for you.

Passing the energy ball

When you feel ready, slowly pass the energy ball to someone sitting next to you and place it gently in their hands, making the sort of hand movements that you might make when passing a big cupped handful of the lightest feathers from you to another person: you are passing something light and delicate and leaving it gently in their hands.

They will be holding their hands together, palms cupped, ready to receive the precious ball from you.

As you place the ball in their hands and release it, what do they experience? Many people can notice pressure, heaviness, or fizzing; sensations vary.

Can that person now build up and intensify this energy ball and then pass it back to you? What do you experience?

Explore intent

Reiki is very simple. It follows your thoughts; it follows your focus. Where you direct your attention is where the energy goes, whether you are focusing your attention on someone in front of you on a treatment table, or whether you are focusing on someone who is 1,000 miles away.

This section is all about demonstrating to you how simple Reiki is, how easily it can be directed, without using complex rituals, and how much effortless control you have over the energy.

You will be going through a number of exercises (I recommend you spend a few weeks on these exercises) and you will need to find people to practice on – in person and at a distance – if you are going to get the most out of this section.

What will I be doing?

Remember to carry out Kenyoku and Joshin Kokkyu ho every day: your baseline Reiki practice, though if you already know about and are practising "Hatsurei ho" then just keep on with this exercise daily, since it contains Kenyoku and Joshin Kokkyu ho, as you know.

Here are some of the things that you will be doing:

- Sending energy to particular parts of someone else's body using intent
- Sending energy across a room 'using your eyes'
- Sending energy across a room using direct intent
- Radiating Reiki out of your whole body
- Carrying out distant healing using intent only
- Focusing energy within yourself using intent

We have been teaching these methods on our live and home study courses for many years now, and these approaches seem to work for most people.

I wish you an exciting journey with this section of the book. Follow the instructions; get lots of practice (that's the key to it really), and you will be surprised by what is possible!

Have fun!

By the way, I recommend that you keep notes on your experiences as you progress through this section, so you can look back and review your progress.

Treatment couch exercises

Here you are going to be working on other people, discovering that you can move energy through someone else's body, and direct the energy to a particular part of someone's body, using visualisation, using intent (they are the same thing).

I recommend that you carry out these exercises on people who have already been attuned to Reiki because they will probably be more sensitive to the energy and its movements and they will be able to give you better feedback than people who have not been attuned.

I am going to describe these exercises:

- Sending energy along someone's leg
- Enveloping someone's head with energy
- Moving energy from one part of the body to another

I suggest that you carry out these exercises on a few different people, to obtain a range of responses. If you just practise on one person, you might just by chance be working with a person who has no sensitivity to energy and will not be able to give you any useful feedback.

If you practise on more people, you increase the likelihood of finding people who can feel stuff happening and feed their experiences back to you.

'Many hands' exercise

The recipient lies on the treatment table face-up. You are going to be resting your hands, one over the other, on top of the nearest knee to you.

Allow the energy to flow for a while, so you are setting up a 'baseline' to compare things with.

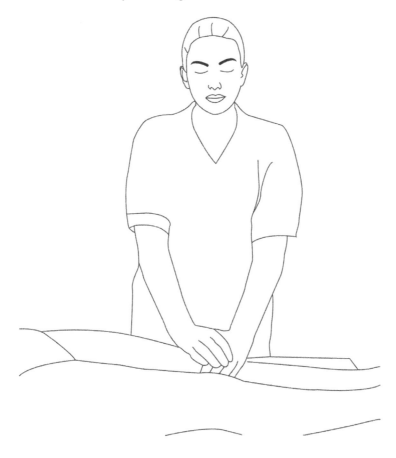

When you are ready, tell the recipient that you will be trying something different now and imagine that you have a couple of sets of extra arms coming down off each shoulder, with additional hands resting on the ankle/foot, on the upper thigh, and in other treatment positions.

Have in mind that energy is flowing out of all the sets of hands – real hands and imaginary hands – into all the different treatment positions; keep the energy flowing.

(In this image, slightly confusingly I realise with hindsight, extra hands have been 'placed' along the opposite upper leg)

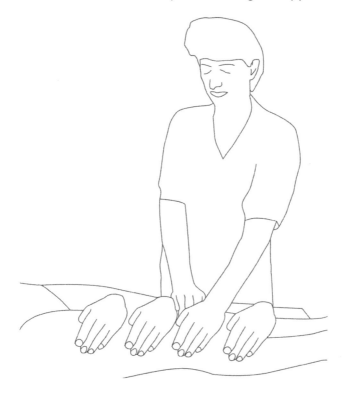

After several minutes, obtain some feedback from the recipient.

Most people will notice that the heat/tingling/heaviness etc that they felt in the knee has 'spread out' to cover a wider area of their leg, sometimes filling the whole leg with energy. Occasionally even the other leg 'comes out in sympathy' to an extent.

A few people might be aware of exactly where the 'imaginary hands' were placed, which is very interesting because, of course, they had no idea what you were visualising and where the additional hands were resting.

What you have done is to direct energy using visualisation. The exercises would have worked just as well if you had just used disembodied hands resting in those different treatment positions.

The visualisation is just a convenient shortcut that focuses your intent, focuses your attention in a particular way.

In fact the exercise will also work if you simply allow your attention to rest or to dwell in those different places, over a wider area: the energy follows your thoughts and focuses itself where you are focusing your attention.

'Enveloping the head'

The recipient lies on the treatment table face-up. You are going to be resting your hands on either side of the recipient's head, by the temples, without touching.

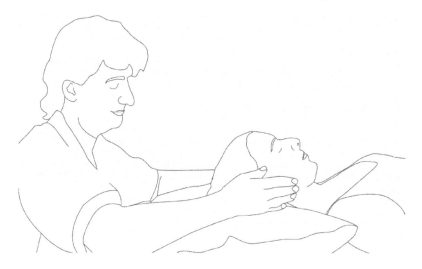

Allow the energy to flow for a while, so you are setting up a 'baseline' to compare things with.

When you are ready, tell the recipient that you will be trying something different now and imagine that you have a couple of pairs of hands cupping around the back of the head and hovering over the front of the face (see photographs overleaf) as well.

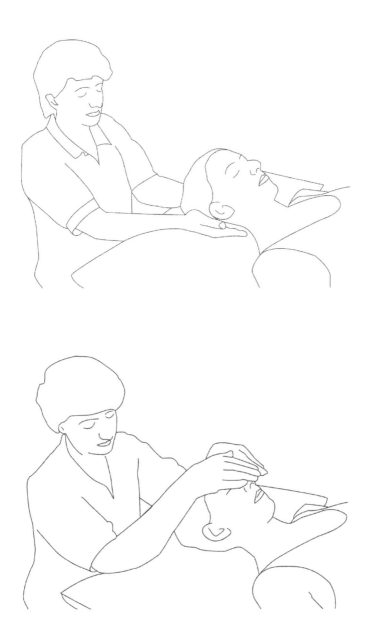

Imagine that energy is flooding into the back of the head, into the front of the face, as well as the temples, surrounding the head with energy. Allow the energy to flow for a little while as you maintain this visualisation.

Tell the recipient that things will be changing now, and dissolve the visualisation; take your attention away from the head, perhaps look out a window or into the distance, and just allow the energy to flow through your hands for a while.

Time for round two: when you are ready, tell the recipient that you will be trying something different again now and imagine that you have a couple of pairs of hands cupping around the back of the head and hovering over the front of the face, as before.

Imagine that energy is flooding into the back of the head, into the front of the face, as well as the temples, surrounding the head with energy.

Allow the energy to flow for a little while as you maintain this visualisation.

After several minutes, obtain some feedback from the recipient.

Most people will notice that the sensation in their head changes quite considerably when the additional imaginary hands are introduced, and that the sensation dies away quite a lot in between the two 'enveloping the head' sessions that you carry out.

What you have done is to direct energy using visualisation. The visualisation is just a convenient shortcut that focuses your intent, focuses your attention in a particular way.

Moving energy from head to foot

The recipient lies on the treatment table face-up. You are going to be resting your hands on the person's shoulders.

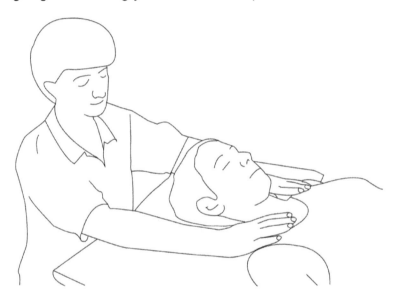

Focus the energy, focus your attention, on their head in general.

You could imagine that energy is flooding out of your hands into their shoulders, whereupon the energy makes the journey through their body into their head, or you could just focus your attention on their head itself and imagine that this is where the energy is focusing itself, irrespective of where your hands are.

The energy remains and envelops them and builds there. Keep that energy flowing for a little while.

When you are ready, tell the recipient that you will be trying something different now and take your attention away from the head completely.

While keeping your hands on the shoulders, direct your attention towards the recipient's right foot/leg: focus your attention on their lower leg and foot and imagine that energy is flooding through their body to build up and accumulate in the leg.

Allow the energy to flow there for a few minutes.

Then bring your attention back to the head and focus on channelling energy to the head for a few minutes.

Finally, obtain some feedback from the recipient.

Most people will notice the sensation in their head and that the sensation dies away quite a lot, to be replaced by an awareness of heaviness or heat or tingling or coolness in the lower leg, with this then dissipating and the sensations coming back to the head again.

What you have done is to direct energy using visualisation. The visualisation is just a convenient shortcut that focuses your intent, focuses your attention in a particular way.

Remember to take notes on what you experience when you carry out these exercises.

Sending Reiki across a room

Here you are going to be practising sending Reiki to someone using your eyes, and then going through an exercise where you will discover that you didn't need to use your eyes after all!

We recommend that you carry out these exercises on people who have already been attuned to Reiki, because they will be more sensitive to the energy and its movements and they will be able to give you better feedback than people who have not been attuned.

If you just work on non-attuned guinea pigs you may be disappointed by the responses that you receive.

I suggest that you carry out these exercises on a few different people, to obtain a range of responses.

Sending "with your Eyes"

The recipient sits the other side of the room from you, with their eyes closed. They have their eyes closed because they are more likely to notice or experience the energy that you send them.

You are going to be sending three separate 'blasts' of Reiki to their forehead; you will send the energy to their forehead because they are more likely to experience the energy strongly there than if you sent it to another part of their body.

Look down at the ground, to make sure that you are not sending by mistake.

When you are ready to send the energy with your eyes, look at the forehead and say out loud "sending". You do this so that the recipient can tie in their experience with when you say that you are sending – and not sending – the energy.

To send Reiki with your eyes, look with a loving state of being, defocus your eyes and stare straight through their forehead, imagining that the energy passes with your gaze. Keep the energy flowing for, say, 15 seconds.

When you are about to stop, say out loud "looking away" and take your attention away from the forehead and look at the floor.

After a 5-10 seconds, send a further blast of Reiki in the same way, and then a further blast.

Obtain feedback from the recipient.

If you would like to experiment further, now repeat the experiment, but this time you will send the energy to a different part of the recipient's body. The results are likely to be less consistent than with the 'forehead' example, but should still work for many people.

This technique is simply a practical example of intent. You are using the "eyes" ritual as a way of focusing your intent in a particular way, in this case sending the energy to someone's forehead. This method will work just as well even if you are not 'sending with your eyes', and we will experiment with this shortly.

Sending Reiki using intent

The recipient sits the other side of the room from you, with their eyes closed, as before. But this time, instead of staring at them and sending Reiki with your eyes, you are going to be sitting with your eyes closed too.

You are going to be sending three separate blasts of Reiki to the recipient's forehead, and you are going to do this by simply focusing your attention on their forehead in your mind's eye and imagining that the energy is focusing itself there, concentrating itself there, for about 10-15 seconds.

When you send the energy, say out loud "sending", and when you have taken your attention away from the forehead, say "not sending".

Repeat three times.

Obtain feedback from the recipient.

You should find that the recipient will be as much aware of the receipt of energy as when you were sending "with your eyes". The important thing here is your intent, your attention: you focused your attention on the forehead and the energy followed your thoughts and focused itself there.

Remember to take notes on what you experience when you carry out these exercises.

Flooding Reiki out of you

Here you are going to be practising sending Reiki out of your entire body, flooding it from yourself to another person in order to produce effects on a mental/emotional level.

We recommend that you carry out this exercise on people who have already been attuned to Reiki, because they should be more sensitive to the energy and its effects and they may be able to give you better feedback than people who have not been attuned.

But if you don't have any Reiki to hand to practise on, by all means practise on non-Reiki-attuned volunteers and they may well give you all the feedback you need.

We suggest that you carry out these exercises on a few different people, to obtain a range of responses.

"Radiating" Reiki

The recipient sits the other side of the room from you, with their eyes closed. They have their eyes closed because they are less distracted this way and because they are more likely to be aware of the effects of the energy that you send them.

You now have to ask the recipient to think about a difficult or sad event in their lives, connecting with some of the thoughts and emotions that they would have felt at that time, making themselves feel thoroughly miserable, basically!

After a couple of minutes, let the recipient know that you are going to be doing something now.

What you do is this: sitting with your eyes closed and your hands in your lap, simply feel that you are 'connecting' with the other person's thoughts and emotions. Intend that Reiki is radiating out of your body, flooding towards the other person, surrounding and engulfing them with energy.

Keep on sending the energy for a few minutes.

Obtain feedback from the recipient.

Most recipients feel unable to continue focusing on the sad event in their life. Their reactions can vary: some people forget what it was that they were focusing on, others find that the situation is resolved now, so they don't really feel bad about it anymore, others find that the situation is being 'walled up' by a layer of white mist, so they cannot direct their attention on the past event any longer… and it no longer makes them sad.

All this can be done while you are just sitting there (and of course you can use this technique with your eyes open too).

Remember to take notes on what you experience when you carry out these exercises.

Distant healing exercises

Here you are going to be practising carrying out distant healing without using any symbol or set ritual.

If you are thinking nice warm thoughts about someone, then *dzzzzt* … you have just sent distant healing to that person, you have sent them Reiki because you were focusing your attention on them and Reiki follows what you are focusing on. You have already discovered this for yourself when carrying out the exercises in previous stages, and distant healing is no different: where you focus your attention is where the energy focuses itself.

This concept would obviously cause problems for people who believe that you should not send Reiki to people without getting their permission first.

They would have to make sure that they only *thought* about a person if they obtained their permission first!

We recommend that you carry out this exercise on people who have already been attuned to Reiki, because they should be more sensitive to the energy and its effects and they may be able to give you better feedback than people who have not been attuned.

But if you don't have any Reiki to hand to practise on, by all means practise on non-Reiki-attuned volunteers and they may well give you all the feedback you need.

We suggest that you carry out these exercises on a few different people, to obtain a range of responses.

Distant Healing Using Intent Only

Arrange with your recipient for them to sit down in a quiet room with no distractions, ready to receive Reiki from you at the time you agree upon.

When it comes to the allotted time, close your eyes, focus your attention on the recipient, feel yourself merging with them, becoming one with them, and allow the energy to flow for maybe 5 minutes. Just 'be' with the energy, 'be' with the other person, merge with them and allow the energy to flow.

Distant Healing to a specific area

Arrange with your recipient for them to sit down in a quiet room with no distractions, ready to receive Reiki from you at the time you agree upon.

When it comes to the allotted time, close your eyes, focus your attention on the recipient, feel yourself merging with them, becoming one with them. Focus your attention on a particular part of their body: either an area that you decided upon beforehand, or an area that comes to mind when you 'merge' with them. Focus the energy there for several minutes. Let the energy flow.

Then focus the energy onto another area of their body, again either an area that you decided upon beforehand or an area that comes to mind as you are sending the energy. Focus the energy there for several minutes. Let the energy flow.

In both of these examples, obtain feedback from the recipient.

"Remote Treatments"

Since you can make a simple connection with another person at a distance using intent, and since you can direct the energy to various parts of their body using visualisation/intent, then why not try experimenting with doing a full treatment on someone at a distance.

This is not distant healing – where you are sending Reiki in a very general way - because you are actually directly connecting to, focusing on, and engaging with the other person for an extended period of time, say 40 minutes.

This takes quite a lot of concentration, even though for chunks of time you will be merging with the energy and just 'drifting'.

You can sense their energy and direct the energy intuitively.

Start with the shoulders, and follow a series of hand positions, finishing with the ankles maybe, just like a 'live' treatment, but directing the energy into different positions using visualisation/intent.

Remote scanning

I want to expand a little on my comment that you can "sense their energy" because once you have made a distant connection with your volunteer, you can if you wish carry out a form of distant 'scanning'.

What you do is to sense in your hands the different amounts of energy that would be flowing through your hands into the recipient were you carrying out 'real' scanning on them, while they were resting on a treatment table in front of you.

There are two ways of doing this, either using a prop of some sort (say a teddy bear) or just closing your eyes and using pure intent/intuition.

If you use a prop, lay a teddy bear (or a pillow to represent the recipient's body) in front of you. Hover your hands above the prop, as if you were scanning it, and make that distant connection to the recipient. Move your hand slowly from one place to another, over the prop's 'head' or 'torso' or 'legs' and notice how the sensations of energy in your hand changes from one place to another: you are sensing their energy needs.

If not using a prop, just close your eyes and hover your hand or hands in mid air, ready to 'scan'. Make your distant connection to the recipient and in your imagination move imaginary hands from one place to another over their body.

You do not move your real hands: they just hover in a convenient position.

As your attention moves from one part of your distant recipient's body to another, be aware of how the sensations in your hand changes. Where are the intense areas?

Remember to take notes on what you experience when you carry out these exercises.

Hands-on Self-Treatments

This exercise is all about demonstrating to you that you are able to move the energy, or focus the energy within yourself, in much the same way that you moved and focused the energy when you were practising on other people earlier in this self-help programme.

if you are doing a hands-on self-treatment and you cannot get your hands into a position so that they can rest on the part you want to treat, then you can just intend/imagine that your hands are resting on the chosen area, or imagine that the energy is flowing to that area.

Try treating your back without touching

Try this experiment: lie on your back on your bed. You are going to treat your back but you are not going to rest your hands on your back.

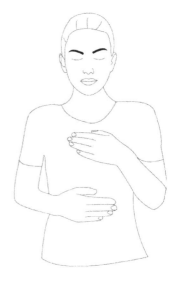

Simply rest both your hands on your abdomen, or heart and solar plexus, and intend that the energy flows from your hands to the back

It will do that, and your back may heat up as if there were hot water bottles underneath you!

Hands-off Self-Treatments

Now let's take this one stage further: if you are able to send energy to another person in the same room as you, without using your hands, and if you are able to send Reiki to someone by way of distance healing, even to a particular part of their body at a distance, then of course you can focus the energy on yourself using intent/visualisation, without your hands having to enter into the process at all.

Try this experiment: lie on your back on your bed, or sit in a comfortable chair. Imagine that you are drawing energy down to you from above, and you are going to focus your attention on, you are going to concentrate the energy on these areas for a few minutes each:

1. Forehead
2. Temples
3. Right shoulder
4. Heart
5. Solar Plexus
6. Left hip
7. Right ankle

Where you focus your attention is where the energy is going to flow.

What happens? Where do you feel the energy, how does it feel and how do the sensations change in your body as your attention moves from one place to another?

Treating Organs & Chakras

Now of course if you can focus the energy on various parts of your body using intent/visualisation then there is no reason why you can't be quite specific when doing this, for example by focusing the energy on various body organs or on particular chakras.

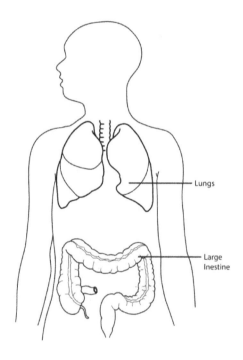

Within Taoism there is a practice referred to as "The Inner Smile" where you focus warm thoughts and compassionate feelings towards various internal organs, like your Liver, Spleen, Small Intestine, Lungs etc.

If we did this as a Reiki person, the energy would follow our focus and direct itself on the organs that held our attention.

In Traditional Chinese Medicine (TCM) the 'organs' are seen as energy fields that are represented not just by physical organs in the body, but also by states of mind and emotions, so by working on your Liver and Gall Bladder, for example, you are also working on the emotion of anger and the state of mind of 'Planning' (Liver) and 'Decision-making' (Gall Bladder).

You can read about this in a lot more detail in my book, "Five Element Reiki".

Working on your elements

On the Reiki Evolution web site you can download my "Reiki Inner Smile" meditation, which talks you through the entire process or treating your Wood, Fire, Earth, Metal and Water elements.

Working on your chakras

Visualise your root Chakra and imagine Reiki focusing there. Allow the energy to dwell there for a few minutes before moving on to the next Chakra. Treat all seven of them.

In my Reiki blog, search for "chakra meditation" and you can find a free Chakra meditation to follow, which has a bit of a Reiki Evolution "twist"!

Develop your
intuition

You are already intuitive.

You may not realise it yet, and you may not have too much evidence yet, but you are already intuitive, that is without doubt.

For example, you already know just the right combination of hand positions to use on each person you treat, you already know where the areas of need are, whether they are in front of you or 100 miles away, and you already know just the right amount of time to spend in each hand position.

But at the moment you may not be able to access that intuitive information, the intuition that is already there. Your conscious mind is sitting there like a great big lump, getting in the way and preventing you from accessing what is already within you.

So learning to work intuitively is all about learning to get your conscious mind out of the way, and trusting what comes to you, trusting what you perceive. Working intuitively is all about getting your head out of the way, suspending your disbelief, and allowing it to happen.

To work intuitively you need to not try – it won't work if you *try* - you need to simply be there with the energy, merge with the energy, and be an observer.

So this section is all about giving you different opportunities to get your mind out of the way, helping you to not try, helping you to merge with the energy, helping you to suspend your disbelief and let it happen... in different ways.

These exercises will not work for you unless you have a group of people available to you to be willing guinea pigs for your intuitive exercises.

- You will learn to cultivate the right state of mind to attract intuitive impressions.
- You will learn to allow your hands to drift with the energy so that "invisible magnets" pull them to the right place to treat.
- You will learn how to use visualisation in different ways to access intuitive knowledge.

Now, the state of mind that you need to cultivate to allow for intuitive working is also the best state of mind to have when practising Reiki, when giving treatments, when carrying out distance healing, when working on yourself.

So these exercises will also help you to develop your ability as a channel and your effectiveness as a practitioner.

We have found that Reiki treatments based on intuitive hand positions do something really special for the recipient, more than if they received treatments based on standard hand positions.

Intuitive treatments seem to allow the energy to penetrate more deeply, to produce effects that are more relevant or more profound.

This makes sense because you are directing the energy into just the right combination of positions for them on that occasion.

So from one treatment to another with the same person, you will use different combinations of hand positions, as their energy needs change from one session to another.

We have been teaching these intuitive methods on live and home study courses for years now, and these approaches seem to work for everyone.

I wish you an exciting journey with these exercises.

Cultivating your State of Mind

To do this you are going to be doing some exercises by yourself every day, and you will be practising with other people too.

Solo Exercise

Do this exercise for ten minutes each day.

Make yourself comfortable and rest your hands in your lap. Close your eyes. Take a few long deep breaths.

Imagine energy flooding down to you from above, into your crown, and the energy flows down the centre of your body to your Tanden. Feel/imagine the energy building in your Tanden.

A continuous flood of energy keeps pouring through your crown into your Tanden, where it builds.

As the energy floods through you, feel yourself disappearing into the energy and merging with it, imagine yourself becoming one with the energy.

Just be there with the energy, allowing it to flow. No expectations. Just merge with the energy. This is the state that you will be cultivating as you progress through this course.

Exercise using Guinea Pigs

Do this exercise for about five minutes or so for each person you practise on. It doesn't take very long. Practise on as many people as you can.

The recipient sits in a chair or lies on a treatment couch. It doesn't matter which.

Sit near the recipient.

Make yourself comfortable and rest your hands in your lap. Close your eyes. Take a few long deep breaths.

Imagine energy flooding down to you from above, into your crown, and the energy flows down the centre of your body to your Tanden. Feel/imagine the energy building in your Tanden.

A continuous flood of energy keeps pouring through your crown into your Tanden, where it builds.

As the energy floods through you, feel yourself disappearing into the energy and merging with it, imagine yourself becoming one with the energy.

Just be there with the energy, allowing it to flow.

No expectations.

Just merge with the energy for a minute or so.

Now, in your mind, focus your attention on the recipient. Feel yourself merging with them, becoming one with them. Merge with them for a while.

Open your eyes and look at the person with a feeling of gentle compassion, with no expectations.

- Do you feel drawn to a particular area or areas of their body?
- Is your attention being pulled towards an area?
- Allow your eyes to drift across their body; do your eyes want to dwell on a particular area?
- Do you feel a physical pull towards a particular area?
- Do you have a sense of 'knowing' where the energy needs to go?
- Does a particular word, phrase or image come to mind?
- Do you notice a new sensation or emotion in your body?

In this exercise, you are not using your logical or rational mind: you are not trying to work out a puzzle or try and guess something based on what you can see of the person before you.

You are empty and you have merged with the recipient and you are allowing yourself to resonate with that person, and in doing so you are echoing their state to an extent. This allows you to discover something about their energy needs or their thoughts or their emotion.

Simply accept what comes to you without filtering it or doubting it in any way; be a neutral observer.

Letting the energy guide your hands

In this section you are going to start to practise an 'intuitive method' that has come from Japanese style Reiki, and was first taught in the West by Frank Arjava Petter and Hiroshi Doi.

We teach this method on Reiki Evolution Second Degree courses and it works very well for most people within a very short space of time. In fact, students are often very surprised by how effortless the whole process can be.

The technique helps you to 'stop trying'.

Exercise with your volunteer in a chair

This exercise is ideal for using on people where you don't have the time or opportunity to set up or use a treatment couch. All you need is a chair.

Your volunteers do not need to be Reiki-attuned: they can be anyone. You are not particularly looking for feedback from them, and your main priority is to practise allowing the energy to guide you, to allow your intuition to come through.

Do this exercise for about 10-15 minutes or so for each person you practise on. It doesn't take very long. Practise on as many people as you can, so you can experience the pull of different energy fields and for people with different energy needs.

How to perform "Reiji ho"

The recipient sits in a straight-backed chair and you stand behind them or to one side of them.

Make yourself comfortable and bring your hands into the prayer position. Close your eyes.

Take a few long deep breaths to calm yourself and to still your mind.

Imagine energy flooding down to you from above, into your crown, and the energy flows down the centre of your body to your Tanden. Feel/imagine the energy building in your Tanden.

A continuous flood of energy keeps pouring through your crown into your Tanden, where it builds.

As the energy floods through you, feel yourself disappearing into the energy and merging with it, imagine yourself becoming one with the energy.

Just be there with the energy, allowing it to flow. You have no expectations: just merge with the energy for a minute or so.

Now, in your mind, focus your attention on the recipient. Feel yourself merging with them, becoming one with them. Merge with them for a little while.

After a few moments, bring your hands (which are in the prayer position) up so they rest against your forehead, and say silently to yourself "please let me be guided"... "please let my hands be guided" ... " show me where to treat".

Move your hands down and apart so that they are hovering near the recipient's head in a neutral, comfortable position. Your hands and arms are loose, there is no resistance; your hands will drift smoothly and easily.

Imagine the energy is flooding through you: into your crown, through your arms and out of your hands. Feel yourself disappearing into the energy, merging with the energy, becoming one with the energy... and allow your hands to drift.

There is no resistance; your hands will drift and glide smoothly and easily.

Allow your hands to drift

That's all you do: allow it to happen.

As you do this you may notice a gentle or subtle pull on your hands. Allow them to drift until they come to rest. It can feel like your hands are sliding across slippery ice, so there is no resistance.

You may now have a feeling that your hands are in the 'right' place, and you may feel a lot of energy flowing through your hands. You may feel that you are 'locked' in place.

Allow that energy to flow for a minute.

Now bring your hands back to your 'start' position, with your hands apart and hovering in a comfortable position, and repeat the process. You are practising allowing your hands to drift with the energy; you are not practising treating someone at the moment.

Keep on moving your hands back into the start position, and allow them to drift to where they want to go.

NOTE

- Sometimes both hands will drift and come to a stop, and on other occasions only one hand will move
- Sometimes a hand will drift further away from the body, or move closer to the body. In the latter case do look to see where your hand is going!
- Sometimes a hand will not come to rest, but will keep moving in an interesting 'energy dance'. Just go with the flow and accept what happens as the right thing for the recipient on that occasion

Ask for feedback

Although this exercise is more about practising intuitive working, it can be useful and helpful if your volunteer lets you have some feedback about what they experienced.

Ask them what they noticed, what sensations they had.

If you felt a strong pull to one area in particular, mention that and they might be able to tell you about, for example, an injury or a recent headache that might explain why your hands were drawn to a particular area.

Remember, though that Reiki works on all levels, so there may not be an obvious explanation for why your hands were attracted to a particular area.

Reiki works on mental states, it works on emotions, in works on the spiritual level, it deals with stuff that is long gone but there's still a trace that needs to be dealt with, and it deals with stuff that is 'on the boil' and hasn't manifested yet as a particular problem.

So don't try to puzzle out why!

Using Reiji ho in practice

In practice, wherever your hands come to rest, you would rest your hands on the person to treat, obviously depending on the part of the body your hands are hovering over: some areas should be treated with the hands hovering above the body, not resting on the surface, for the sake of propriety.

Reiki is basically a hands-on treatment technique, and Reiji ho does not change that. There is something very special and particularly healing about compassionate human touch.

Reiji ho shows you where to rest your hands down to treat... unless you are moved to place your hands further away from the body, in which case you are being guided to channel energy into a layer of the aura for a time.

You may find that after a while, the hand that seemed to be hovering in the aura then moves closer to the body, and may repeatedly move away and towards the body, before moving on elsewhere.

Have no expectations.

Let the energy guide you.

Couch "Reiji ho" Practice

In this section, you will be going through essentially the same process as before but your volunteer will be lying on a treatment couch and you will be practising "Reiji ho" while standing at different locations around the treatment table.

In this way, you can become familiar with the sort of 'pull' that you might experience when working on the head and shoulders, when standing by the torso or pelvis area, when standing by the legs and when standing at the foot of the table.

You are still not treating the recipient: you are using this time to practise opening to the energy and being neutral and empty, with no expectations.

The instructions below are basically the same as what I outlined in the previous section but I think they bear repeating, to help you to become familiar with the process.

Do this exercise for about 15 minutes or so for each person you practise on. It doesn't take very long. Practise on as many people as you can.

What to do

The recipient lies on a treatment couch and you stand beside their torso.

Make yourself comfortable and bring your hands into the prayer position. Close your eyes. Take a few long deep breaths.

Imagine energy flooding down to you from above, into your crown, and the energy flows down the centre of your body to your Tanden. Feel/imagine the energy building in your Tanden. A continuous flood of energy keeps pouring through your crown into your Tanden, where it builds.

As the energy floods through you, feel yourself disappearing into the energy and merging with it, imagine yourself becoming one with the energy. Just be there with the energy, allowing it to flow. No expectations. Just merge with the energy for a minute or so.

Now, in your mind, focus your attention on the recipient. Feel yourself merging with them, becoming one with them. Merge with them for a little while.

After a few moments, bring your hands (which are in the prayer position) up so they rest against your forehead, and say silently to yourself "please let me be guided"... "please let my hands be guided" ... " show me where to treat".

Move your hands down and apart so that they are hovering over the recipient's body in a neutral, comfortable position. Your hands and arms are loose, there is no resistance; your hands will drift smoothly and easily.

Imagine the energy is flooding through you: into your crown, through your arms and out of your hands. Feel yourself disappearing into the energy, merging with the energy, becoming one with the energy... and allow your hands to drift.

As you do this you may notice a gentle or subtle pull on your hands. Allow them to drift until they come to rest. You may now have a feeling that your hands are in the 'right' place, and you may feel a lot of energy flowing through your hands. Allow the energy to flow for a minute.

Now bring your hands back to your 'start' position (whatever position that was) and repeat the process. You are practising allowing your hands to drift with the energy; you are not practising treating someone at the moment.

Keep on moving your hands back into the start position, and allow them to drift to where they want to go.

Now move to another part of the body, so you are standing next to the head and shoulders (at the head of the treatment table), the hips, or the knees, at the foot of the table, and repeat the exercise, each time seeing where your hands want to drift, allowing them to come to rest if they want to, and repeating the process to see if they drift to the same area each time.

Using Reiji ho in practice

In practice, wherever your hands come to rest, you would rest your hands on the person to treat, obviously depending on the part of the body your hands are hovering over: some areas should be treated with the hands hovering above the body, not resting on the surface, for the sake of propriety.

When your hands come to rest you usually find that there is a lot of energy coming through. This makes sense because you have just put your hands in just the right combination of positions for that person on that occasion.

After a while you will notice that the flow of energy subsides, and you know that it is ok to move on to the next combination of hand positions that your intuition suggests. If you move your hands away too soon you will simply be guided back to those positions to treat some more!

In practice you will find that you end up with fewer hand positions than you used when following your 'standard' hand positions.

To start a treatment, what I always do is to treat the shoulders for about 10 minutes to begin with to get the energy flowing and to help the recipient to enter a lovely, peaceful state.

Then I move on to use Reiji ho on the head. Usually I end up with 'non-symmetrical' hand positions.

Then after say 25 minutes I move on to the torso and let the energy guide me there, and I stay in each hand position until I feel that it is right to move on.

Remember to take notes on what you experience when you carry out these exercises.

Finding areas of mental and emotional need

This section is all about developing your intuition a little further. You will be allowing your hands to drift to particular areas of the body: areas of physical need and areas of mental/emotional need.

You will also allow the energy to guide you in terms of how long to spend in each hand position.

Extended Intuitive Practice

Do this exercise for about 20-25 minutes or so for each person you practise on. It doesn't take very long. Practise on as many people as you can.

The recipient lies on a treatment couch and you stand beside them.

Make yourself comfortable and bring your hands into the prayer position. Close your eyes. Take a few long deep breaths. Imagine energy flooding down to you from above, into your crown, and the energy flows down the centre of your body to your Tanden. Feel/imagine the energy building in your Tanden.

A continuous flood of energy keeps pouring through your crown into your Tanden, where it builds.

As the energy floods through you, feel yourself disappearing into the energy and merging with it, imagine yourself becoming one with the energy. Just be there with the energy, allowing it to flow. No expectations. Just merge with the energy for a minute or so.

Now, in your mind, focus your attention on the recipient. Feel yourself merging with them, becoming one with them. Merge with them for a little while.

Seeking areas of physical need

If you like, you can use the procedure where you hold your hands in the prayer position and move them up so they are resting against your forehead, before using the following phrase. Say silently to yourself "please let me be guided to areas of physical need".

Move your hands so that they are hovering over the recipient's torso in a neutral, comfortable position. Your hands and arms are loose, there is no resistance; your hands will drift smoothly and easily.

Imagine the energy is flooding through you: into your crown, through your arms and out of your hands.

Feel yourself disappearing into the energy, merging with the energy, becoming one with the energy… and allow your hands to drift.

There is no resistance; your hands will drift and glide smoothly and easily.

Allow your hands to drift.

As you do this you may notice a gentle or subtle pull on your hands. Allow them to drift until they come to rest. You may now have a feeling that your hands are in the 'right' place, and you may feel a lot of energy flowing through your hands. Allow the energy to flow for a minute.

Now bring your hands back to your 'start' position (whatever position that was) and repeat the process, affirming again "please let me be guided to areas of physical need".

Seeking areas of mental/emotional need

Now repeat the process, but this time affirm "please let me be guided to areas of mental/emotional need".

Now move to another part of the body, so you are standing next to the hips, or the knees, and repeat the exercise, each time seeing where your hands want to drift in terms of physical need, and mental/emotional need.

Intuitively knowing whether to stay or move on

Choose a hand position to use, based on your intuitive practice, and rest your hands on the recipient to treat them

Rest your hands in that position and let the energy flow. You will probably notice quite a lot going on in your hands.

In your mind's eye, imagine that you are moving your hands away from that treatment position.

What do your imaginary hands want to do? Are they happy to drift away from that treatment position, or do they want to move back again, a bit like being pulled by an elastic band perhaps?

Repeat this visualisation every few minutes, and after a while – as the flow of energy subsides – you will notice that the imaginary hands become content to move on elsewhere.

NOTE

These exercises are here to demonstrate to you that you have at your disposal more intuitive information than perhaps you realised.

By setting your intent in a particular way you can be guided to areas requiring a physical healing energy, and those areas that require energy that works on the mental/emotional levels.

You can use the "imaginary hands moving away from their treatment position" whenever you aren't quite sure whether it is yet time to move away from the treatment position you are using. Most of the time this will be clear to you because of what you are feeling in your hands, but sometimes you may not be completely sure.

Use this method to intuit whether to stay there for longer or to move on.

Remember to take notes on what you experience when you carry out these exercises.

Intuit with imaginary hands

In this section you will develop your intuition even further, so that you can intuit the areas that require treatment without having to even hover your hands, or even have the recipient in the same room as you.

You will be allowing imaginary hands to drift to particular areas of the body, with the recipient lying on a treatment couch in front of you, and you will be using your imagination to connect to other people distantly, to intuit areas of need remotely.

Extended Intuitive Practice

Do this exercise for about 10-15 minutes or so for each person you practise on. It doesn't take very long. Practise on as many people as you can.

The recipient lies on a treatment couch and you stand beside them.

Make yourself comfortable and bring your hands into the prayer position. Close your eyes. Take a few long deep breaths. Imagine energy flooding down to you from above, into your crown, and the energy flows down the centre of your body to your Tanden. Feel/imagine the energy building in your Tanden.

A continuous flood of energy keeps pouring through your crown into your Tanden, where it builds.

As the energy floods through you, feel yourself disappearing into the energy and merging with it, imagine yourself becoming one with the energy. Just be there with the energy, allowing it to flow. No expectations. Just merge with the energy for a minute or so.

Now, in your mind, focus your attention on the recipient. Feel yourself merging with them, becoming one with them. Merge with them for a little while.

Say silently to yourself "please let me be guided"… "please let my hands be guided" … " show me where to treat".

Keeping your hands in the prayer position, I want you to imagine that you have a pair of imaginary hands hovering over the person. In your mind's eye, see where the imaginary hands want to drift.

Allow the imaginary hands to come to rest, and when they have stopped moving, bring them back to their starting position and see where they want to drift now.

Now bring out your real hands and hover them over the person. See where they drift.

Now move to another part of the body, so you are standing next to the hips, or the knees, and repeat the exercise, each time starting with your hands in the prayer position, merging with the energy, allowing your imaginary hands to drift a few times, and then bringing in your real hands to see where they want to drift.

Keep on repeating this sequence: use imaginary hands and then notice what your real hands want to do.

Remote Intuitive Practice

This exercise can be done on your own, sitting quietly in a room with your eyes closed and your hands resting in your lap. Connect to the energy and feel yourself merging with the energy.

Focus your attention on another person, someone who is not near you, and feel yourself merging with them. In your mind's eye, imagine them standing in front of you.

Bring out your imaginary hands and hover them over the person in your mind's eye. Look to see where the imaginary hands want to drift. When they come to rest, bring them back to the starting position and repeat.

Because you are doing this in your imagination, you can be creative: rotate them by 180 degrees so that you can intuit areas of need on their back. Zoom in like a telephoto lens to look in more detail, using smaller imaginary hands that can be guided precisely to one spot.

Play around with this and see what you can perceive. Maybe what you have perceived makes sense in terms of what is going on with the person you were practising on.

NOTE

These exercises are here to demonstrate to you that you have at your disposal more intuitive information than perhaps you realised.

The muscle movements that guided your hands were just a 'tool', a way of accessing intuitive information in a concrete or physical way, rather like dowsing using a pendulum.

You can access this intuitive information using visualisation too, as you have just discovered.

Distance is no barrier to the use of this method either, and in fact if you were to imagine in your mind's eye that you were treating the person, focusing the energy into the imaginary hand positions that you intuited, then you will be sending distant healing to them and focusing the energy into the areas you visualise.

If you don't visualise too well at the moment, you can focus your attention on the recipient in a different way: instead of 'seeing' them, become aware of them in a physical way and notice where their bodies seem to want to 'pull' the energy.

Imagine that you are moving your way through or feeling your way through their body and notice physical qualities that draw your attention towards a particular area.

Remember to take notes on what you experience when you carry out these exercises.

My prescription for intuitive success

I hope that this section has opened your eyes to some of the intuitive possibilities that there are within the Reiki system, and I hope that you now have a strong belief that you are intuitive.

If you routinely use Reiji ho when you treat, you will find that your hands move more quickly and consistently, and that the process becomes effortless.

Allow your hands to drift, and treat when they come to rest (though sometimes they will keep drifting: just go with the flow and let them do what they want). Stay in the hand position until you feel it is time to move on, using the simple intuitive check if you're not quite sure whether to stay or to move on.

Usually it will be quite clear to you.

As well as allowing us to enter into a lovely blissful 'merged' state when treating, a wonderful meditation, Reiji ho does something really special for the recipient too.

By getting your conscious mind out of the way and allowing the energy to guide you, you are allowing the energy to flow strongly through you and directing the energy into just the right combination of hand positions for them on that occasion.

Use hypnotic suggestions

You might know that I trained as a Cognitive Hypnotherapist and NLP Master Practitioner with the Quest Institute at Regent's University and I have used my knowledge and experience of creating hypnotic suggestion patterns to create a series of Guided Reiki Meditations that combine the gentle power of Reiki with the potency of Ericksonian hypnosis.

Hypnotic suggestions can be very powerful on their own, of course, but I have discovered that when combined with Reiki they become particularly effective, as if the Reiki is in some way used as a 'carrier' to powerfully embed the suggestions in your subconscious mind.

Interestingly, Frank Arjava Petter, author of several books about Japanese style Reiki, and Hiroshi Doi, member of the Usui Reiki Ryoho Gakkai (Usui memorial society) describe a couple of techniques called Seiheki Chiryo and Nentatsu ho, both of which involve sending a thought or a positive affirmation into yourself or into a client, using Reiki as a way of helping to embed a useful idea or behaviour change.

Seiheki Chiryo means 'habit treatment technique' and Nentatsu Ho means 'send a thought technique'.

So using positive affirmations, or carefully-crafted suggestions, along with Reiki acting as some sort of a 'booster', has quite a good pedigree in the West and in the East!

I put together three collections of unique Reiki Guided Meditations which I tested extensively on a large group of Reiki volunteers they work fantastically well, and in fact they surpassed my expectations. It seems that when gentle suggestion patterns are combined with Reiki meditations, a very powerful combination is created, helping the listener to move powerfully in a new better direction.

The collection that you will probably be most interested in at the moment deals with Mindfulness, Energy Sensitivity and Developing Intuition.

I recommend that you listen to the 'developing intuition' track every day (the track lasts for about 12 minutes) for 4-6 weeks, during which time the beneficial changes develop and solidify.

It's powerful stuff.

The Nentatsu Ho Meditations can be found on the Reiki Evolution web site for immediate download:

www.reiki-evolution.co.uk

Develop your intuition further

You are already intuitive and I think you probably know that by now.

If you have worked through the previous section - Develop Your Intuition - you will be using the "Reiji ho" method comfortably and confidently when you work on someone else, allowing your hands to drift with the energy to the right places to treat.

You have learned to get your conscious mind out of the way, you have learned to not think, not try, you have learned to merge with the energy with no expectations, and to allow your hands to drift.

You have learned to cultivate an 'open' state of mind that makes you receptive to intuitive knowledge, and you have practised merging with the recipient when you treat them.

Not only that, but you will also have discovered that you can focus your intuition selectively, to be drawn to areas of physical need, or mental-emotional need, and that you can also intuit areas of need at a distance, without the recipient having to be there in front of you on the treatment couch.

Now we are going to take things further, by showing you that you are able to perceive a great deal about what is going on with your energy system and the energy system of the people you work on. You will be flexing your intuitive 'muscles' in different ways and discovering what is possible for you.

In this section you will find many exercises and for a lot of them you will need to find willing volunteers. Take your time and enjoy experimenting.

Monitoring the State of Your Chakras

We are going to move on to something that I find exciting: being able to intuit the state of your chakras: to discover:

- Which old too much energy, or are spinning too quickly
- Which hold too little energy, or are closed to an extent or spinning sluggishly
- Which seem just fine

You may not realise it just yet, but you already know the state of your chakras. All the information and insights that you need are already there, within you.

As we go through the exercises described in this section of the book, you may be able to access these insights really easily and effortlessly or you may need to practise before you feel comfortable with trusting what is coming to you.

Intuitive knowledge can come to people in a whole range of different ways. For some, they just 'know' what their chakras are doing. For others, the information pops up in one of many different forms: a word, a sound, a feeling or an image.

Some people need a bit more 'structure' in order to access what is already within them, and they can use different 'props'. A prop might be a weight dangling on a string or some other 'already set up beforehand' physical movement.

A prop can also involve using a visual image in your mind's eye, where they w ay that the image changes or moves or presents itself provides you with the information that you need.

'In your head' ways of accessing intuitive knowledge are usually more speedy and versatile than physical-based methods.

For example, if you're using a pendulum you have to keep on opening your eyes, picking it up and putting it down, whereas if you're doing it all 'in your head' then you can perceive the state of your elements in real time, instantly, 'on the fly'.

Your Goal

Your goal should be to end up able to sense the state of your chakras without having to resort to a physical prop, though they can be useful to begin with to help build your confidence and to give you an opportunity to practise being in an 'accessing intuition' state of mind.

You will find lots of different options and variations described below. Try them out and see what works best for you. Every time you try one you are practising getting your head into the right sort of state to access what you already know on some level.

Why chakras?

People reading this who trained with Reiki Evolution may be surprised to find me talking about chakras because we don't tend to really focus on or mention chakras a great deal on Reiki Evolution courses.

Chakras are talked about on most Reiki courses and this is because Reiki has travelled alongside, or within, the New Age movement in the West for many years and has assimilated a lot of New Age preoccupations, like spirit guides, crystals, Angels and, of course, Chakras.

There is nothing wrong with thinking about or working with Chakras but they were not part of the original system that Mikao Usui taught and they have nothing to do with Reiki really, other than that they are one way of viewing the human energy system.

But people are familiar with them, a lot of Reiki people will probably have read books about them and their associations, and they are a useful 'target' for practising intuiting stuff.

 So we will intuit our chakras because they are a simple set of energy centres that we can focus our attention on.

And if you are interested in flexing your intuitive muscles further, in my book "Five Element Reiki" you will find out how to use intuitive approaches to discern the state of your Elements (Wood, Fire, Earth, Metal and Water).

The Five Elements are a fascinating subject.

General impressions: an "inner knowing"

A simple method for opening to intuition

Let's start with a simple opening-to-intuition meditation and we can find out what your subconscious is going to provide you with.

This is what you can do:

Sit quietly with your eyes closed and take a long, deep breath. Imagine any stress or tension just drifting out of you as you exhale.

Be still.

Remind yourself of your connection to the energy through your crown and imagine energy flooding down to you from above, through the centre of your body to your Tanden.

Feel or imagine the energy building up and becoming more intense in your Tanden. Imagine yourself filling with energy. Feel yourself merging with the energy.

Now focus your attention on your Root Chakra; you know where this is in your body. Be still with this Chakra and be aware of any impressions that you might have.

Maybe you might have a word come to mind, or a phrase (which you might hear inside your head as a voice) or a feeling, an image of some sort, an image of a word or an "inner knowing" or understanding about the state of this Chakra.

- Does it spinning too quickly at the moment?

- Is its energy depleted in some way? Is it closed to an extent or is it spinning sluggishly?

- Or does it seem fine, balanced, perfectly appropriate for you?

Take your time. Make a note of what impression you have: too much, too little, or just fine.

Then move on to the Navel Chakra.

Move through the other Chakras – Solar Plexus, Heart, Throat, Third Eye and Crown - making notes on your impressions each time.

You may find that the state of the Chakras is quite clear to you straight away; if so, congratulations! It can be surprising sometimes how quick, how immediate the response can be: as soon as you ask the question, the answer is there!

It doesn't have to be difficult.

Or you might find that this takes a bit of practice, and what you are practising is tuning into yourself, noticing your energies, how they feel, their strength or weakness or 'just-fine'-ness.

What happened during these exercises?

Were your impressions coming through to you in a fairly standard way, with a particular word or image or sensation or feeling each time, or did it seem quite random?

You might find that your subconscious mind has showed you, through this exercise, its 'default' way of displaying or providing the information to you. You shouldn't put up any barriers or expect your intuition to come to you in any particular way.

Try this exercise later on, and on a different day, and see what happens.

What did you experience?

You may be surprised to find that you have perceived the Chakras as having quite distinct characteristics compared to each other, and you may have a strong feeling about which Chakras seem fine, which Chakras require some attention, and which ones need boosting rather than restraining.

You may notice that the Chakras are not all nice and even and the same size, yet your impression is that this is the correct 'presentation' for them, that it is ok for a particular Chakra to be bigger or more prominent.

We should not assume that everyone's Chakras should all be the same as everyone else's; we can accept how they are and accept our impression of which Chakras require our attention.

Intuiting the state of someone else's Chakras

You know more than you realise about the state of your energy system, and that of other people.

You *know* what is going on with your Chakra system; you *know* what is going on with the Chakra system of other people.

To access this intuitive information you need to focus your attention in a particular way, and be open to receive intuitive impressions.

Here is a suitable process to go through, while sitting in the same room as someone who has volunteered to be a test subject for you:

Sit quietly with your eyes closed and take a long, deep breath. Imagine any stress or tension just drifting out of you as you exhale.

Be still.

Remind yourself of your connection to the energy through your crown and imagine energy flooding down to you from above, through the centre of your body to your Tanden.

Feel or imagine the energy building up and becoming more intense in your Tanden. Imagine yourself filling with energy. Feel yourself merging with the energy.

Now focus your attention on the other person.

Imagine your energy expanding to engulf the other person. Feel yourself merging with the other person, becoming one with them.

Consider their chakras; be aware of their chakras. Have no expectations of what you may experience.

How do they seem to you?

Is your attention pulled towards one or some of them?

Maybe you might consider each one in turn, and compare it with the next; maybe you will have an overview, and then focus on one or a few in particular.

Do they seem balanced, or do they seem not quite right somehow; in what way?

Do this for maybe 5 minutes and then withdraw your attention back to you; withdraw the energy back to you.

Make notes on what you experience; maybe repeat the process on another occasion, so you can compare. Has anything changed in the intervening period?

Intuiting Chakras at a distance

Of course, the distance between you and the recipient is immaterial and this exercise will work just as well whether your volunteer is sitting next to you, in a nearby room or building, or 10,000 miles away.

For Reiki, distance is irrelevant.

Dowsing - General

If you are going to treat yourself, it will be useful if you can see the effect of the self-treatments on your elemental imbalances from day to day. A simple and effective way of doing this is by dowsing: using a pendulum.

When the pendulum moves, it is moving because you are jiggling it: it still has to obey the rules of physics! It is moving because of your muscle movements, because of nervous impulses from your brain, and the movements are controlled not by your conscious mind but by your subconscious mind… but it is still you that is moving it.

Some people get on well with dowsing right away, while for others it can take practice and perseverance before it will work consistently for them. The best state of mind to have when dowsing is that of being neutral and empty, simply interested in seeing what movements it makes, rather than 'cheerleading' or pushing for a particular response, which will not give you useful results since it is possible to force an outcome.

Not everyone gets on well with a pendulum, but it's a useful skill to have if it 'clicks' with you, and you can use it as a stepping-off point, to build your confidence in your intuitive ability and to get you use to 'tuning in' to your intuition, before going freestyle and intuiting purely in your head.

In this section I'm going to talk about using a pendulum in general – the basic principles – and then I move on to show you how to use a pendulum to look at the state of your elements in quite a precise way.

Introduction

Pendulums can be purchased inexpensively. I have a nice brass pendulum on a metal chain; you can use other metal or crystal pendulums too. Basically they need to have some weight to them and be able to dangle freely on a chain or a thread.

'Yes' and 'No' Answers

The first thing to do is to find out how your pendulum is going to interact with you: what movements it is going to make for different responses.

You need to know what it is going to do to show you a 'yes' or 'no' answer. Try asking 'am I a man?' or 'am I a woman?'

Blank your mind for a few moments, hold the pendulum away from your body, suspending it between your thumb tip and index fingertip, relax, and see what it does.

Don't rest your elbow on your leg or the arm of a chair because the pendulum won't give you a strong response: your muscles need room to move it!

For me, 'yes' is a clockwise movement and 'no' is side-to-side, but it seems to vary from one person to another.
You could try saying 'show me your yes response' and 'show me your no response' and see what happens.

If you try asking 'what should I do now' then you may elicit a response that means ' I can't answer that question with a yes/no', or 'that is a stupid question'.

This is a useful response to have, actually, since otherwise you are limiting the pendulum to a 'yes' or 'no' response, neither of which may always be the appropriate answer!

You can interpret the 'stupid question' response as meaning 'you need to re-phrase your question before I can answer it properly'.

The 'Neutral' position

I have found that it is easier for the pendulum to give you answers quickly if it is already moving, rather than holding it still every time, whereupon it has overcome inertia every time it answers you.

In my case, I continually swing the pendulum forwards-and-backwards as a 'neutral' position before asking the questions, because that motion is different from my 'yes', 'no' and 'stupid question' responses.

Obtaining 'Permission'

Various books recommend that you ask a few questions before entering upon a new endeavour, as follows:

1. Can I do this? (Am I able to do this?)
2. Should I do this? (Is it right or appropriate for me to do this?)
3. May I do this? (simply politeness really)

If you get 'yes' responses to all the questions then you can go ahead.

If any of the answers are 'no' then do not try any more at that time. You do not have to go through this procedure every time you use a pendulum, only when you are intending to use a pendulum in a different way, or for a different purpose, than you have before.

Dowsing Chakras

Dowsing the state of someone's chakras is not something that you do when carrying out Five Element Reiki, and not something that you need to do when practising standard Reiki, but it is a useful exercise to carry out in order develop your skills with the pendulum.

Ask 'am I able to use this pendulum to dowse the state of a person's chakras?' If you get a 'yes' response then you can ask these questions:

- What will you show me if the chakra is open?
- What will you show me if the chakra is closed or spinning sluggishly?
- What will you show me if the chakra is spinning too fast?

For me, the responses are my 'yes', 'no' and 'stupid question' responses.

If you were going to experiment on yourself, just sit quietly and focus your attention on your crown chakra. Get your pendulum moving (if you have a convenient 'neutral' movement) and say to yourself 'show me the state of my crown chakra'; see what the pendulum does. Then move on to the third eye, throat etc. all the way to the root chakra.

Do this on different days and notice if there are any changes. You are just flexing your intuitive 'muscles', getting used to clicking into a receptive state of mind.

If you are experimenting on someone that you are going to be treating, and they are lying on a treatment table, do this: before you start the treatment, hold the pendulum so that it dangles over the crown chakra, say to yourself 'show me the state of the crown chakra', and see what the pendulum does.

Then move on to the third eye, throat etc. all the way to the root chakra.

Make a note and then repeat the process at the end of the treatment to see what difference there is.

In fact you do not have to dangle the pendulum over each chakra; you can happily dowse the chakras standing by the person's side.

You do not have to have the subject in the same room as you, either, so you can dowse the state of their chakras before they arrive for the appointment!

Within the world of dowsing, it is common for the dowser to have some sort of 'witness' - for example a lock of the person's hair, by way of making a definite connection with the person about whom they are seeking information.
I have not felt the need to do this with Reiki clients, so I believe that Reiki and intent is connection enough.

Common Chakra 'presentations'

I have found that it is quite common for the throat, heart and solar plexus chakras to be closed, which ties in with inability to express oneself and current/long term emotional issues respectively.

I found a closed root chakra in a girl with anorexia and a woman with multiple addictions.

I found fast-spinning third eye chakras in a counsellor, research chemist, a molecular geneticist and web consultant.

Chakra changes over time

It seems to me that the Chakras do not flap open and shut from one moment to the next, but reflect a general trend within the individual over recent periods of time of variable length, so you are unlikely to see an immediate transformation in their 'Chakra profile' from one treatment to another.

However, sometimes an individual Chakra can change from one treatment to another, going from being closed to being open, going from being fast-spinning to being more restrained, and occasionally a Chakra can become closed when it has previously been open, though this is only temporary.

Using the pendulum to look at the state of the Chakras gives you an insight into what is going on in the person at an energetic level, and usually reflects what the person has been telling you about their problem, or gives you a better understanding of what they are experiencing.

Interestingly, changes in the Chakra profile can also tie in with the changes that a person reports during a course of treatments, so you can see what is going on underneath, and the differences that these changes produce on the surface.

What to do if you forget to bring your pendulum

On occasion I have forgotten my pendulum by accident, and used an 'imaginary' one instead.

I have held my hand in the usual 'holding a pendulum' position, imagined that I had the usual weight dangling from my fingertips and noticed what movements my arm muscles have made my hand produce.

Although some people believe that the pendulum moves of its own accord, quite separate from the person holding, I don't believe this. Your arm muscles move the pendulum: that's why it jiggles. And your unconscious mind generates the muscle-movements.

With practice, and as you allow your unconscious mind to control the movements, they can become quite pronounced and easy to notice. And with practice you may find that you start to know what the pendulum is going to do, before it does it! Then it's time to move beyond the use of any sort of a pendulum.

Other uses during Treatments

Try using a pendulum to obtain advice about which symbol's energy to channel during the treatment you are about to carry out, or to see if you need to carry out a gentle introductory treatment that excludes the use of symbols.

Try asking the pendulum whether the patient needs to come back for another treatment.

Other Questions to ask

Some people use pendulums as a form of 'kinesiology', to find out about any vitamin or mineral deficiencies that they may have, or any food allergies or sensitivities.

Try asking these questions about yourself: hold an item of foodstuff and say to yourself "Is it healthy for my body for me to eat this".

See what happens.

Book recommendation

Most books on pendulums and dowsing seem very preoccupied with finding underground watercourses and mineral deposits!

I can recommend this now out-of-print book, though:

"Anyone Can Dowse for Better Health"
Arthur Bailey, Quantum Books 1999

Intuit with an imaginary pendulum

Using a pendulum, using muscle movements, isn't the only way of accessing intuitive knowledge. We can use creative visualisation to access our intuition, and this can be quicker than using a 'prop' and waiting for muscle movements to jiggle a crystal on a string.

Introducing your imaginary pendulum

We have just been talking about using a pendulum, so let's try using an imaginary one!

You might be surprised how straightforward it is for you to move from a real pendulum to an imagined one because the intuitive information that you are accessing is just the same; you are just altering a little bit the method that your subconscious is using to present it to you.

So, bring out your imaginary pendulum in your mind's eye and notice how it appears to you, its size and shape, length and weight, its density or physical 'presence'. You do nothing with your hands: this is entirely a mental exercise.

Practise moving your pendulum in different ways: front and back, side to side, clockwise, anti-clockwise. Feel its 'density'.

Because this is a new pendulum for you, you need to start by obtaining 'permission' to use the pendulum (see "Dowsing –

general" above) and ask questions to establish what its 'yes', 'no' and 'stupid question' responses will be.

Don't assume that your imaginary pendulum is going to move in the same way as the physical one you have been using.

This is a new pendulum!

Play around with this and see what's possible for you.

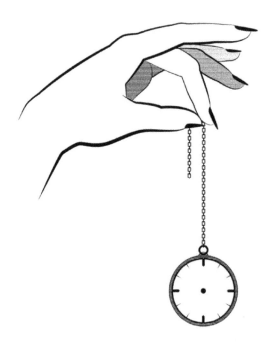

Intuit using imagined text

OK, let's move away from things that are swinging, whether for real or in our imaginations, and let's take a look at things that might just pop up in your mind's eye.

An intuitive method that works well for some people is to use words, written out in one's imagination, and notice what happens to those words and what meaning that might convey to us.

Try bringing up in front of you images of the words for the seven chakras. Look at these words:

Root
Navel
Solar Plexus
Heart
Throat
Third Eye
Crown

Intend that these words represent the state of your chakras.

Maybe you don't see the words in a vertical list. Maybe you see them spread out horizontally, or written on cards that look a bit like playing cards. Maybe they are written on little flags, or stones, maybe they are hovering in the air above some sort of surface. Who knows how they will appear!

It doesn't matter how they appear to you: just accept what comes to you.

Now look at each word in turn, or you might notice one or two that just jump out at you straight away.

You might notice that one word stands out as **larger**,

or in **bold type**, or in a *different font* or in a **different colour**.

One word might be smaller than the rest.

Interpreting what comes to you

The chakra or chakras that stand out like this are the ones that need your attention.

Maybe you can't see a different font or size, or boldness... but maybe one of the words is buzzing or jumping up and down or is in a different colour, maybe a word is flashing on and off or seems so much heavier than the others, while another word wants to sail off like a helium balloon.

I do not know what your word images will do to indicate the state of a chakra, so you will need to experiment and discover for yourself what your personal 'code' is.

Can you tell whether a chakra is spinning too fast or too slowly, by the way its word appears to you?

Compare the results of this way of intuiting with the results that you get from using a real or imagined pendulum.

How do they compare?

Intuit using an imaginary 'slider'

You can obtain the same answers that a pendulum might give you by using a constructed visual image, something that you bring to existence in your mind's eye.

What I like to use is an imaginary 'slider'. You have probably seen sliders in photos of recording studios, where they have banks of dozens of them on mixing desks, controlling volume and other effects

You can bring into your mind's eye a single sliding scale, either running horizontally or vertically. I use them vertically because that's how they look in real life. I find sliders to be really versatile. You may find that too, or you may not like them.

So, here you can see a vertical scale. Imagine that at the top of the scale lies the answer 'yes' and at the bottom lies the answer 'no'.

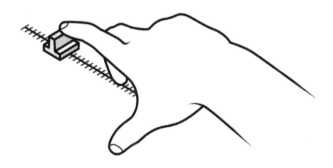

Imagine that the slider is at the very middle point of the scale to begin with.

Ask a question and see where the slider goes: to the top or the bottom. If the slider stays in the middle, maybe vibrating or jiggling in an uncertain fashion, that means that it is unable to answer the question, or you need to rephrase the question somewhat.

You can use this slider in exactly the same way that you can use a real or imagined pendulum, obtaining a 'yes' answer, a 'no' answer and a "I can't answer that question" response.

And if you think about it, this isn't really a great deal different from the "imaginary hands" that you experimented with when you were practising "Reiji ho" earlier.

There you experienced your intuition in terms of imagined hands that drifted with the energy to the right places to treat, in the same way that your real hands would have drifted with the energy.

Here we don't use imaginary hands, but just some other imagined thing, that can move and drift in your mind's eye to show you something that you already know.

And we can also use this sort of visualisation to be very precise about intuiting the state of our chakras.

Here's how…

Looking at a chakra's slider

Bring up the slider and intend that it represents the state of, say, your Root chakra. Say to yourself, "show me the state of my Root Chakra".

Look at the slider. It will probably do one of three things:

1. It stays half way up, perhaps with a little reassuring 'click': the Chakra is ok.
2. It slides down the scale: the Chakra is closed down or spinning sluggishly to the extent that the slider moved down the scale
3. It moves up the scale: the Chakra is spinning faster, to the extent that the slider moves up the scale.

Make a note of this, and move on to the next Chakra.

If you wanted to be precise then you could imagine that there is a 'scale' that runs from +100 at the top, through zero in the middle, down to -100 at the bottom. If you were to do that then you could directly compare the degree of excess and deficiency of the Chakras by using numbers:

Root +50   Navel -20   Solar Plexus +90
… and so on.

You could then compare the numbers from one Reiki treatment to another.

And of course this will work just as well when you are focusing your attention on someone else's energy system.

Intuit using an imaginary 'Mixing Desk'

If you get on well with the idea of a 'slider, you might also get on well with this, which is to use an imaginary 'mixing desk' like they have in a recording studio, with seven different sliders, and you can see a cartoon of something like that here:

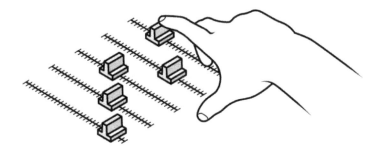

Each slider has a little knob that slides up and down the vertical track. One slider is for each Chakra, arranged from left to right in this order: Root, Navel, Solar Plexus, Heart, Throat, Third Eye and Crown.

As before, if the slider is at the very top of its track then it represents a very fast-spinning Chakra (and perhaps you might interpret this as +100). If the slider is at the very bottom of its track then this represents a slow moving or closed Chakra (and perhaps you might interpret this as -100).

If the slider is smack bang in the middle of its track, and you could imagine a little 'click' sound as it rests there, then the scale is at zero: the Chakra is in balance.

Using the mixing desk in practice

Using seven sliders next door to each other...

1. Bring into your mind's eye an image of the 'mixing desk' with its seven sliders, going from left to right displaying Root, Navel, Solar Plexus, Heart, Throat, Third Eye and Crown, one slider for each Chakra.
2. Say "Show me the state of my Root Chakra".
3. See what happens to the first slider on the left.
4. If it stays where it is and does not move, maybe making a little clicking sound, then that Chakra is in balance. If it slides up then the Chakra is spinning too fast. If it slides down then the Chakra is spinning sluggishly or closed down. The distance it travels shows you the amount of the excess or deficiency. You could even 'zoom in' in your mind's eye and imagine 10% increments, like a thermometer scale. Where does the slider stop? What is the figure?
5. Write it down.
6. Now move on to the next slider, the one for the Navel Chakra. The slider starts on the 'balance' point, half way up. See where it slides; see where it stops. What is the figure?
7. Now follow this procedure for the other Chakras: Solar Plexus, Heart, Throat, Third Eye and Crown.

Using Physical Movements to Intuit your Chakras

Not everyone gets on well with visualising things, though it has to be said that you don't need to be able to visualise things very well: even a fuzzy, dim image works perfectly well; images don't have to be in perfect focus or in Technicolor!

In fact, a lot of people who think that they 'don't visualise very well' don't realise how badly everyone else is visualising things!

Visual memory and visual images are a bit like the images that cameras on the first mobile 'phones produced: grainy and a bit rubbish!

In any case, not being able to visualise, or worrying about whether you can visualise well enough, won't hold you back in terms of intuition because you can use physical versions of the visual images if you like.

I shall explain.

If you have trained with Reiki Evolution at Second Degree, you will be familiar with 'Reiji ho', the intuitive method where you allow the energy to move your hands, which drift with the energy to the right place to treat.

You have already been practising this approach if you worked through the exercises in the "Develop Your Intuition" section of this book.

When practising Reiji ho, most people find that it doesn't take very long before the energy starts to move their hands (or, rather, you allow the energy to guide your hands, because you are in control of this process at all times).

In fact, sometimes people find that the energy causes their hands to drift away from the body, sometimes quite a distance, to say 1-2 feet away, where they are being guided to channel the energy into the aura for a while.

So you know that the energy, or your intuition or your subconscious mind, is able to control muscles and direct movements of your hands and arms, if you allow it to.

Your physical slider

Imagine that you are holding a credit card between your thumb and bent index finger – the card is horizontal – rather like you were just about to slide the card into the slot in a cash machine.

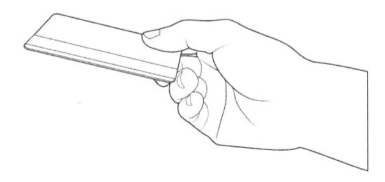

Alternatively, you can imagine that you are holding a pen or conductor's baton between your thumb and index finger:.

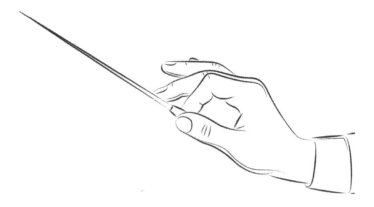

Either of these is your physical 'slider'.

You are going to imagine that there is a vertical scale that your hand/slider can move up and down. You start with your hand in what seems like is the middle of the scale: a comfortable position to hold.

Say to the slider "please slide to the top of the scale"; your hand should move upwards and then stop (mine moves up by about 9 inches).

Then return the slider to its centre 'stop' and ask the slider to slide down to the bottom of the scale; your hand should move downwards and then stop.

If the slider moves ridiculously far up and down, (or moves along an unhelpfully-small distance, for that matter) just tell it that it is too long or too short and show it, by moving your hand, where the top and bottom points should be.

Now you have your physical slider which you can use instead of imagining a visual image.

You can also use your slider in two ways:

As a 'yes/no' scale

This is rather like dowsing with a pendulum. "YES" is at the top of the scale, "NO" is at the bottom, and if the slider hovers in the middle then it can't answer your question in a YES/NO fashion.

As a graduated scale

Here you can have +100 at the top, -100 at the bottom and 0% at the centre point of the scale.

Start with the slider at that centre point, half way along the scale.

A question like, "show me the state of my Heart Chakra" will cause the slider to move up or down the scale to the relevant percentage, to show whether the Chakra is balanced, spinning too quickly or too slowly.

Exploring a chakra's levels

Having discovered that you are able to perceive someone's Chakras in various ways, why not try delving deeper into someone's Chakras to see if you can perceive which aspect of a particular Chakra is in need of attention?

If you know that, say, their Root Chakra is in need of attention because it is spinning too quickly or is closed down to an extent, which aspect of the Chakra is in greatest need of your attention?

Is it the physical aspect? Is it the mental/emotional aspect? Is it the spiritual aspect of this Chakra that needs attention?

There are various ways of finding out this information:

1. Let the information come to you
2. Use a pendulum
3. Use an imaginary pendulum
4. Use imagined text
5. Use an imaginary slider

Let the information come to you

Sit quietly with your eyes closed and take a long, deep breath. Imagine any stress or tension just drifting out of you as you exhale. Be still.

Now focus your attention on your Root Chakra; you know where this is in your body. Be still with the Chakra and be aware of any impressions that you might have.

Maybe you might have a word come to mind, or a feeling, an image of some word or an "inner knowing" about the state of this Chakra.

What aspect of this Chakra require the most attention? Or does no aspect of the Chakra require any more attention than the others? Take your time.

Make a note of what impression you have: physical, mental/emotional, spiritual... or no greater need for any aspect.

Use a pendulum

You can use the pendulum to give you YES/NO answers about the Chakra. A useful first question to ask would be, "Is any aspect of this Chakra in greater need of attention than any other?"

If NO, there's no need to ask anything more.

If YES, you need to find out which aspect (physical, mental/emotional, spiritual) needs most attention.

Ask, "Does the physical aspect of this Chakra have the greatest need of attention?"

Carry on asking, as necessary, until you find out which aspect has the greatest need.

Use a pendulum with a dowsing grid

Here's another idea. Instead of YES/NO answers, use a dowsing grid. On this grid there are three locations: one for Physical, one for Mental/Emotional and one for Spiritual.

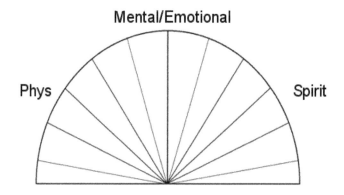

This is what you do:

1. Hold the pendulum with its point hovering over the midpoint of the baseline, the point from which the 'spokes' radiate, or set it moving along horizontally, in 'neutral'.
2. Say "Which aspect of the Root Chakra is in greatest need of attention".
3. See in what direction the pendulum swings.

If the pendulum swings horizontally, side to side, then no aspect of the Chakra has the greatest need of attention.

If the pendulum swings towards the word "Spirit", that aspect is in greatest need. If it swings up and down the page, the Mental/Emotional aspect is in greatest need. If the pendulum swings towards the word "Phys" then that aspect is in greatest need.

Make a note, and move on to the next Chakra that seems out of balance.

Use an imaginary pendulum

Obviously, anything you can do with a real pendulum, you can do with an imaginary pendulum, which you read about earlier. If you get on well with an imagined pendulum, use that instead in the above couple of examples.

Use imagined text

We spoke earlier about how to use imagined text to bring your attention towards a particular Chakra or Chakras that need attention. Now we can use the same approach to see if any aspect of an unbalanced Chakra requires your attention.

Layout some words in front of you, in whatever way they want to display themselves:

Physical   Mental/Emotional   Spiritual

Notice if any of these words attract your attention in any way, through how they look or how they behave. If one word stands out, that is the aspect that requires your attention. If none stand out, no aspect has a greater need.

Use an imaginary slider

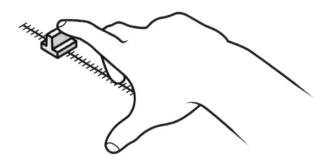

Now let's look at this using an imaginary slider. You can set up the slider so that the bottom of the scale represents the physical aspect, half way up represents the mental/emotional, and the very top of the scale represents the spiritual aspect.

Focus your attention on the Chakra you are interested in and allow the slider to move to the appropriate level. What will happen if there is no aspect in particular that requires extra attention? Who knows? You'll have to find out for yourself!

Maybe the slider will slowly b from one end to another, fall off its guide rail and fall down a hole or disappear in a puff of smoke! Let your unconscious mind show you.

What to do with this information

The whole point of intuiting areas of need for yourself and for the person you are treating, other than the fact that you are flexing your intuitive muscles and rendering yourself effortlessly intuitive through repeated practice… is that you use the information to guide where you direct the energy, when treating yourself or your client.

So having determined which areas of yourself need attention, you can now focus Reiki on those areas by resting your hands on or near them, and/or using intent/visualisation.

For example, you can focus the energy on a particular Chakra by resting your hand or hands near it and/or by focusing your attention on that Chakra.

You may have an impression of which symbol to use, if any, when treating the Chakra, or you may have intuited specifically which aspect of the Chakra has the greatest need.

To focus on the physical aspect you would use energy from CKR, which elicits earth ki. To focus on thoughts and emotions you would use energy from SHK, which elicits heavenly ki.

To focus on spiritual aspects you could use the Usui Master Symbol or imagine that you are channelling very high frequency energy, suitable for producing balance at that rarefied level.

I have used the Chakras as an example in a lot of these exercises even though they didn't really feature in the original system that Mikao Usui was teaching.

This is partly because they are well-known within the world of Reiki, because of the way that Reiki travelled within the New Age movement for many years, and incorporated a lot of New Age principles and preoccupations, for example Chakras, Angels, Crystals, Spirit Guides and the like, during that time.

Also, there are endless books about the associations of the Chakras, and they are straightforward to access and intuit!

In my book, "Five Element Reiki", you would find that all the intuitive activity is directed towards determining what imbalances there are in someone's elements: Wood, Fire, Earth, Metal and Water.

Over the next few pages, you are going to see a variety of approaches that you can use to discover areas that need treating, in yourself and in other people, that are unrelated to the chakras, and the point of these exercises, again, is that once you have discovered an area of need, you can then do something about it by resting your hand or hands on or near that area, and/or focusing your anntion on that area so that the energy flows there.

Hope that makes sense.

Internal scanning by flooding with light

This is another visual exercise that can be used to discern which areas of yourself require attention. Imagine that you are flooding yourself with white light, or golden light, and imagine the body filling up with this light, just like water fills a vessel.

If you notice any areas where the body does not fill up with light - the liver for example - then this indicates a need for Reiki in that area.

You have scanned your body using your perception focused in a particular way.

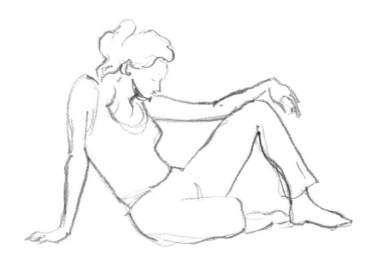

Of course, noticing that there is a need for Reiki to go into your Liver, for example, should not alarm you. You know that Reiki works on many levels so you should not assume that there is some dread disease in your Liver that you just stumbled upon.

Reiki deals with emotional imbalances and mental states and 'spiritual' imbalances as well as physical needs, and you know that in Traditional Chinese Mediicine (TCM) your various body organs hold particular states of mind and emotions.

You also know that Reiki will deal with problems that are now history, but have left some trace that can be dealt with, and will also deal with problems, potential problems, that are currently 'on the boil' and haven't manifested as anything concrete.

So you can just chill, observe the need for Reiki in a particular area, and do something about it, by treating that area and imagining that Reiki is flowing to that place.

Monitoring your healing

And what is interesting is that, as you treat the area, you can at intervals come back to your 'flooding with light' visualisation to see how that area is doing, and notice that as you treat it, light can fill up the area more and more easily, until there is nothing of note there at all.

This may take more than one treatment, of course.

Scanning a client by flooding with light

There is no reason why you can't use this sort of technique with a client if you wanted to. You could sit at the head of the treatment table and rest your hands on the recipient's shoulders, and close your eyes.

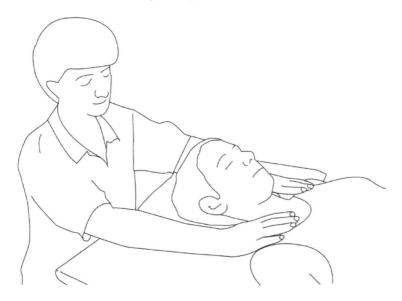

Take a couple of long, deep breaths to calm yourself and to help you to enter a calm, neutral and empty state.

Then what you can do is to visualise white light flooding through the recipient's body from head to foot, emerging out of their feet.

As you do this, you can become aware of any areas where the white light does not want to go, in some way. There may be grey or dark areas or stagnant areas where the light will not flow smoothly and evenly.

Note where they are.

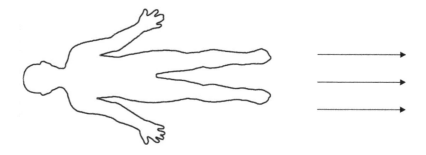

And just as in the previous example, you can use this information to guide your treatment. You can do this in two ways:

Either you can remain sitting at the head of the treatment table, with your hands resting on the shoulders, and focus your attention on those stagnant areas, allowing the energy to follow your focus and flow into those places.

Or during a later part of the treatment, when you are standing by the torso or the legs, you can rest your hands on, or near, those stagnant areas and allow the energy to flow there, perhaps also focusing your attention on the areas if they are within the body rather than on the surface.

Again, you are channelling the energy to the areas upon which your attention is focused.

You flood these areas with Reiki until you start to notice that white light appears to be flowing better and that area has 'smoothed out'.

Please don't talk about dark energy!

When you talk to your client about what you noticed during the treatment (because they always want to know what you 'picked up', don't they?), please do not start talking about "**dark energy**" or negative energy or any phrases like attachments, or even use the word 'stagnation'.

Those words don't really mean anything useful, they are just a way of referring to and interpreting something that is actually unknowable... and it will freak your client out quite unnecessarily if they leave the treatment session believing that they have some sort of dark energy living inside them.

How is that in any way helpful?

Don't do it!

Mapping areas of need

You can play around with this idea in other ways, too. For example, a variation on the 'flooding with light' exercise is one where you bring up a visual image of the recipient's body (or a standardised line drawing of a human body) and look in your mind's eye to see if there are any dark areas, or grey areas, or areas of whatever colour you like, really.

You can do this for yourself and you can do this for a client. Note that the client does not have to be with you, physically, in the room: you can do this remotely if you like.

Just focus your attention on them, feel yourself merging with the energy and with the recipient, and allow your intuition to bubble up to the surface.

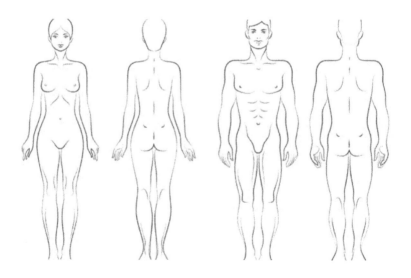

Delving deeper in your body map

You can take this a step further if you like, and 'look' to see where the areas of physical need are, or emotional need, or mental need or spiritual need.

You could look for each aspect on a new, different map, or you might even find that you can see each aspect appearing in a different colour.

Zooming in

Since all this is carried out in your imagination, if you wanted to you could even 'zoom in' and determine precisely where the area of need is.

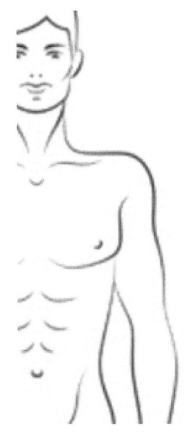

Or perhaps you don't feel this is necessary.

That's fine.

It's useful to experiment, though, to find out what's possible for you.

Experiencing areas of need physically

Now, these examples of course rely on a person being able to visualise to an extent (you don't need to be brilliant at visualising and most people aren't).

It is possible to obtain the same sort of results by imagining that your hands, say, are moving through the recipient's body, in a form of 'scanning', where you focus on the sensations and textures that you can perceive in your fingers and palms.

Travel through the body systematically, noticing where the areas feel soft and smooth, and noticing the areas that feel in some way blocked or constricted, rough or grainy, heavy or sluggish. These are the areas of need.

You can do this for yourself too.

And don't tell a client that they have 'blocks' or 'blockages'. It's not helpful. It's not friendly. It's not nice.

Create bespoke symbols

Introduction

Reiki Synthesis is primarily about using bespoke symbols for yourself and for your clients, and there is a question about the use of symbols that needs to be addressed first.

The question is this: "If Reiki is intelligent and knows where to go and what to do, why do we need symbols?"

Well, we don't 'need' symbols, in that they are not an essential part of Reiki practice, but they are useful because they allow us to frame the energy in a certain way, narrowing the focus of the energy and in doing so increasing the power or intensity of what we are doing, rather like focusing a magnifying glass or a laser.

So, for example, by using CKR we emphasise earth ki and boost the flow of energy, by using one of Taggart's 'Five Element Reiki' symbols we focus the energy intensely on the Wood element, or Water.

And if we are working intuitively – letting the energy or the recipient guide us in terms of which symbol we might use rather than trying to plan and 'work out' what might be best to use – then we are working in partnership with the energy.

Symbols and their energies

You will be familiar by now with the characteristic energies of CKR and SHK, which elicit the energies of earth ki and heavenly ki.

You will have meditated on these energies and you will know how they feel when you are using them.

If you are a Reiki Evolution RMT then you will have been 'attuned' to these symbols on your RMT course, but before your RMT course you weren't attuned to them, and you were able to use the symbols effectively.

You do not need to be 'attuned' to a symbol for it to work for you: you just need to be connected to Reiki and any symbol will mould or frame the energy in a particular way.

On a recent Reiki Synthesis course, here are some of the words that students used to describe the energies of CKR and SHK:

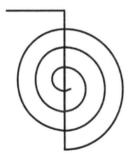 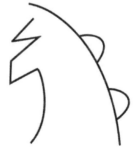

Descriptions of CKR/earth ki	Descriptions of SHK/heavenly ki
Warm	Light
Heavy	Floaty
Weighted	Spacey
Slow	Happy
Downward	A high/a giggle
Grounded	Cold
Swirling	Uplifting
Heartbeat	Upper body
Physical	Elongating
Strong	Airy
Power	Comfy light shoulder blanket
Pulling backwards	Soothing
Gentle	Waves
Engulfing	Awareness of blocked
Vortex	emotions
Solid	Quick energy
Still	Expansive
Present	Still mind
Rooted	'Held'

Some of these words represent people's individual, idiosyncratic experiences of these energies, and some represent a general 'theme', the sort of things that most people say when working with these energies.

How do you experience these energies?

Working with novel symbols

To prove to yourself that symbols that you haven't been attuned to will work effectively in framing the energy, you can do an exercise for yourself.

Take three symbols, for example a circle, a triangle and a square. I am suggesting these because you will definitely not have been 'attuned' to these symbols.

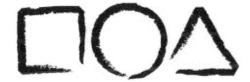

Meditate on the energy of each symbol.

To do that, sit with your hands palms up in your lap and close your eyes. Take a couple of deep breaths to calm yourself and to let go of stress and tension.

Then imagine the symbol up in the air above you. You could imagine it in its entirety, draw it out in your mind's eye or even make physical 'drawing out' movements with your hand, if you like: whatever works best for you.

Imagine Reiki is flooding down to you from the symbol, engulfing you and flowing through you.

For each symbol:

- What do you notice?
- Where do you feel the energy?
- How does it feel?
- How does it make you feel?
- What words or phrases come to mind about the nature of the energy?
- What is its essential characteristic?

You could actually use these symbols to treat someone if you liked, using whichever symbol wanted to be used.

And if you wanted to use a symbol from one of the endless Reiki variations that are in existence (or try it out at least, for yourself and for people that you work on) you can, without having to be specifically 'attuned' to it.

How should you experience these energies?

Well, there is no "should": your own experience is your own experience, and however the energy presents itself to you is the way that you are meant to experience it.

What other people might notice is interesting but irrelevant.

Of course, if you get a big group of people together to carry out this sort of exercise, it is likely that there will probably be some sort of a consensus about how the energy tends to be experienced by most people, but no-one is right and no-one is wrong.

The "Three questions"

How to create a bespoke symbol for yourself

To create a symbol that will frame the energy in a way that perfectly matches your needs, you can use these three questions, which you ask yourself:

1. If the energy that I need in this moment had a shape, what shape would it be?
2. If it had a colour, what colour would it be?
3. If that energy was to be held in a particular part of my body, where would it be held?

Allow the answers to come to you; go with the first thing that comes into your mind. So now you have, say, a green star that needs to reside in your abdomen (I have chosen this randomly). Do this exercise now and draw the symbol, write the colour and write the location below...

Examples of symbols people intuited

Below you can see some images created (intuited) by some of the students who attended my "Reiki Synthesis" course several years ago, to show:

1. The symbol
2. What colour it is
3. Where it should be located

Each student came to the front of the room to draw their symbol on the whiteboard. I am not suggesting that you 'should' receive such an image, colour and location. I am just including them so you can see what came to some people on a live course.

	Location: Heart **Colour:** Shimmering gold
	Location: Heart **Colour:** Green

	Location: Head **Colour:** Cream
	Location: Heart **Colour:** Blue
	Location: Heart **Colour:** Red

	Location: Throat **Colour:** Blue
	Location: Sciatic & various places
	Location: Throat & Third Eye **Colour:** Green

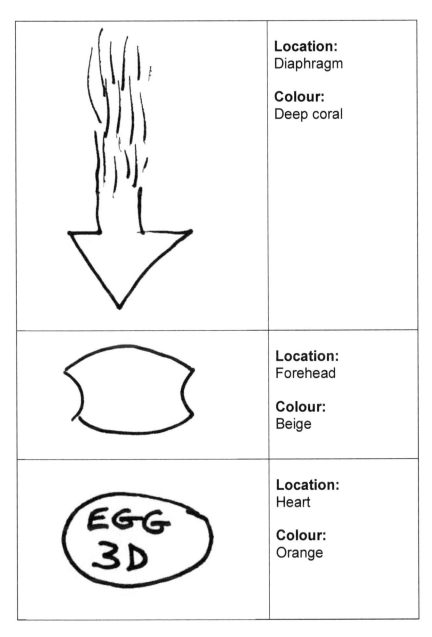

	Location: Diaphragm **Colour:** Deep coral
	Location: Forehead **Colour:** Beige
EGG 3D	**Location:** Heart **Colour:** Orange

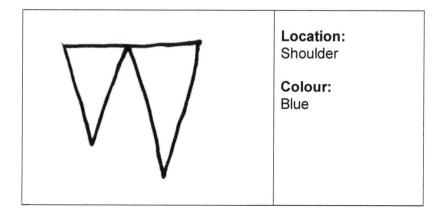

| | Location: Shoulder |
| | Colour: Blue |

Meditate on your bespoke symbol

Imagine that shape in that colour, up in the air above you, representing the source of the energy. This is quite like the symbol meditations that you were introduced to on the Reiki Evolution Second Degree course.

Imagine energy of that colour flooding down to you from the symbol above you, focusing/drawing the energy into that part of your body (in this example, the abdomen).

Feel the energy in that location and allow that colour to flood through your whole body.

Experience that energy for a few minutes.

You could, of you like, imagine that the coloured symbol is actually passing into that location in your body, as that coloured energy continues to flow down to you from that symbol above you.

If you're not so good at visualizing at the moment, focus not so much on the shape of the symbol, but the feel of it, the texture or density: feel the shape rather than seeing it; if you can't see the colour very well, simply intend or 'know' that the shape and the energy has that particular hue.

In doing so, you are embodying the essence of that energy.

As a variation, you might draw the energy to your Tanden as you inhale, breathing the energy to its chosen location on the out-breath; experiment and find out what works best for you.

Adding a fourth question: sound

For those of you who particularly 'resonate" with using sound, or mantras, you could also ask, "If the energy that I need in this moment had a sound, what sound would that be?" and add that sound to your meditation, chanting out loud if you wish.

How to create a bespoke symbol for a client

To use this approach when treating someone, just slightly alter the three questions:

1. If the energy that they need in this moment had a shape, what shape would it be?
2. If it had a colour, what colour would it be?
3. If that energy was to be held in a particular part of their body, where would it be held?

When you treat your client, imagine that colour symbol up in the air above you, representing the source of the energy (you are asking the energy to come to you in a particular 'flavour' that is represented by that coloured symbol).

Draw the coloured energy from that symbol above you, merge with the energy, and channel that colour energy, through your hands, into your client.

Focus your attention on the relevant part of your client's body and rest your hands either on or near that area if you can. Allow the energy to flow there.

Using Reiki as a 'carrier' for particular states

In the above examples we asked for "the energy that I need in this moment", but we can frame our question in a different way, to elicit an energy that provides us with the essence of a particular state or quality that we might want or feel we need.

For example, you might want to embody one of these states:

- Self confidence
- Serenity
- Relaxation
- Peaceful mind
- No mind
- Stillness
- Determination
- Compassion
- Motivation
- Creativity
- Contentment
- Enhanced intuition
- Rejuvenation

What useful or helpful states or qualities could you add to this list? Write some below:

What to ask to elicit the energy for yourself

To elicit such an energy for yourself, just modify the three questions a little, and meditate on or channel the energy (in this example, eliciting creativity):

- If the energy of creativity had a shape, what shape would it be?
- If it had a colour, what colour would it be?
- If that energy was to be held in a particular part of my body, where would it be held?

Do this exercise now and draw the symbol, write the colour and write the location below...

Using an image instead of a symbol

Some people find that instead of a symbol, they have another image come to mind. For example, stillness might be represented for you by the image of a still lake.

If that works for you then go with that, drawing energy from that image in whatever colour and to whatever location you are drawn to.

Meditating on the energy

I have already described above how to "Meditate on your bespoke symbol". Do that now for several minutes and notice how things have changed for you in some way.

What to ask to elicit the energy for another person

To elicit such an energy for another person, use these questions and meditate on or channel the energy into the recipient:

- If the energy of creativity for this person had a shape, what shape would it be?
- If it had a colour, what colour would it be?
- If that energy was to be held in a particular part of their body, where would it be held?

Allow the answers to come to you; go with the first thing that comes into your mind.

So now you have, say, a yellow 2D disc that needs to reside in the client's solar plexus (I have chosen this randomly).

Channelling the energy for someone else

Imagine that shape in that colour, up in the air above you, representing the energy, as you might when using, say, CKR or SHK to treat someone.

Imagine that colour energy flooding down to you from above, flowing through you into the recipient; you focus your attention on that part of their body and imagine the energy/colour/symbol focusing and concentrating itself there.

You might have your hands resting on their shoulders, or you might choose to rest your hands on or near to the part of the body where the energy wants to reside; go with what feels right for you.

How to shift unhelpful emotions

Breathing away unhelpful emotions

Let's just take a pause from the symbol explorations and move sideways into a breathing technique that you can use to help release unhelpful emotions.

We'll come back to symbols later.

If you trained with Reiki Evolution then you will be well used to moving energy in time with your breathing and focusing the energy on particular areas of your body in time with your breathing, for example when carrying out Joshin Kokkyu ho or Seishin toitsu.

If you didn't train with Reiki Evolution but you started at the beginning of this book, you will already be using Joshin Kokkyu ho.

We use this approach in a slightly different way in this section.

What is an 'unhelpful' emotion?

Well, we all have feelings about ourselves or the world that we could usefully let go of in order to move on with our lives in a positive way: sadness, anger, fear, guilt, frustration, shame.

Maybe we have experienced events in our lives that have left their mark, or which bring negative emotions when we think about or dwell on a particular event or situation, or which come to the surface in particular current circumstances.

Maybe we have ongoing negative feelings that return regularly, for example lacking self-confidence, feeling bad about ourselves in some way.

Start by finding the feeling

When we use this technique, we will be using it in short bursts, stopping at regular intervals to see how the feeling has changed.

So before we start, we need to know:

1. Where is the feeling?
2. What is the feeling like?
3. How strong is the feeling?

You need to focus on the feeling to be able to answer those questions.

This may mean that you recall a specific event that gives you a negative feeling, or perhaps you might remember a specific recent situation or event where you have had a negative feeling, perhaps one that occurs often.

Focus your attention on that feeling.

Where is the feeling?

When we have a feeling, we feel it in our body somewhere. We may not be aware of that to begin with, but if we feel something then we can feel it somewhere.

So we can ask a question of ourselves: "If I could feel that feeling in my body, where would I feel it?"

What is the feeling like?

We can focus more intensely on that feeling, and hold onto it more precisely, by asking ourselves some other questions about the feeling:

- "What name does that feeling have?" ...
- "If it had a shape, what shape would it have?"
- "Is that 2D or 3D?"
- "If it had a colour, what colour would it have?"
- "If it had a lightness or heaviness, how does it feel?"
- "If there was a texture, what texture would it have?"

So you might find that you have a dark disc in your abdomen, 3D, quite heavy, with a rough surface, quite dense.

How strong is the feeling?

We need to 'calibrate' the feeling to see how intense it is: "As you focus on that feeling, on a scale of 0 – 10, how strong is it?"

Once we have this information, about the location, characteristics and strength of the feeling, we will then be able to tell when the feeling changes in response to the breathing technique.

We will use the technique for a while and then stop.

We check to see if the feeling has moved, if it seems different in some way, and to see if its strength has reduced.

We are looking for some sort of change. A change is a good sign.

Sometimes a feeling may become more intense but this is not common, and this is by way of 'bringing things to a head' rather than a permanent effect, fortunately!

Using the breathing technique on yourself

You are going to be going through a Reiki breathing exercise that is quite similar to Joshin Kokkyu ho, but instead of drawing the energy into and out of your Tanden, you are going to be moving the energy in different ways, into and out of the location where you have that unhelpful feeling, and by making various 'passes' of the energy through your body.

The idea here is that you are using the energy to disrupt and fragment the energy of the unhelpful feeling, helping it to soften, loosen, disintegrate or dissolve.

You will go through perhaps a couple of dozen breaths and then stop, noticing any changes in how the feeling appears to you or feels, or where it is located, and noticing any changes in its intensity.

You breathe normally and gently.

Do not over-breathe (hyperventilate) because you will get dizzy.

Start by breathing in and out of the feeling where you feel it

Start by imagining that you are breathing in and out of the part of the body where you have the feeling. Get into a nice gentle rhythm.

Acknowledge and thank the feeling

This is an important thing to do.

This feeling is a part of you, a part of you that is doing the best that it can with the resources that it has available. It is not the enemy.

You can have love and compassion for this feeling as it eases itself out of you. Say to yourself, "I acknowledge this feeling and thank it for its contribution".

Add some breathing variations

Here are some variations that you could use when drawing the energy down to you, Joshin Kokkyu ho style:

- Breathe the energy into and out of the feeling
- Breathe the energy into the crown and out of feet
- Breathe the energy into feet and out of the crown
- Breathe the energy into the feeling & out of your whole body
- Breathe the energy into the torso & out of the feeling
- Breathe the energy into the front of body & out of the back of the body
- Breathe the energy into the crown & out of the feeling
- Breathe the energy into the feeling & out of the feet

Follow this sequence

I suggest that you begin by breathing in and out of the feeling (where you feel it) for a few breaths, and then try some variations.

Then return to breathing in and out of the feeling.

Try some more variations, finally returning to breathing in and out of the feeling again.

Now stop and consider the feeling. Focus your attention on it.

1. Is it still in the same place or has it moved?
2. Has it changed shape or colour? Is it still as heavy or dense? What other qualities have changed?
3. How intense is the feeling now, on that scale of 0 − 10?

You should find that the feeling has changed in some way, and has become less strong.

Repeat the breathing exercise and then check again.

The purpose of this exercise is to reduce the feeling to zero on the strength scale, or to a lower level that feels appropriate for you.

For example, if someone is experiencing intense and ongoing grief, they might want to have that feeling reduce but not disappear completely.

What to do when the feeling disappears

When the feeling disappears, you need to test things to see if it has really disappeared.

Try and get the feeling back. Try hard.

You may be able to get the feeling back to an extent, but not as strongly as before; you have drained some of the intensity of that feeling.

Use the breathing method again to reduce this weaker feeling to zero.

Check again: try and get that feeling back. If you can get it back, even a little bit, use the breathing method to reduce it and re-check.

Your aim is to reduce the feeling to zero and to not be able to get it back again.

Working with a feeling on a number of occasions

A negative feeling will not always reduce to zero during one session and that's fine. Some feelings may need to be worked on over a number of occasions before they resolve.

Working with other feelings or beliefs that arise

Occasionally you might find that the feeling you are working on disappears, but when you think of the event associated with that old feeling, a new negative feeling arises.

You can work on the new feeling until it is eliminated.

Occasionally you might find that there is another feeling or belief that is holding you back, perhaps:

- "I can't let this feeling go"
- "I don't want to let this go"
- "This can't resolve as quickly as this" (a belief that change can't happen so quickly)

If you phrase this as a feeling - "I feel like I can't let this go" – then you can work on that feeling, establishing where it is, what it's like, how strong it is, and reducing that to zero using the breathing technique, before returning to deal with what is left of the original negative feeling, no longer held back by that limiting belief/feeling.

Using the breathing method on other people

Using this technique on other people follows the above approach, but we need to tell the client what to do, to explain things and guide them through the process.

Start by finding the feeling

When we use this technique, we will be using it in short bursts, stopping at regular intervals to see how the feeling has changed.

So before we start, we need to know:

1. Where is the feeling?
2. What is the feeling like?
3. How strong is the feeling?

The client needs to focus on the feeling. This may mean that they recall a specific event that gives them a negative feeling, or perhaps they might remember a specific recent situation or event where they have had a negative feeling, perhaps one that occurs often.

Ask them to focus their attention on that feeling.

As before, we ask the client questions to establish where the feeling is, what it's like (how their subconscious mind represents the feeling) and how strong it is, and we re-visit these aspects after each use of the breathing method.

Here are suitable questions

- "As you focus on that feeling, if you could feel that feeling in your body, where would you feel it?"
- "As you focus on that feeling where you feel it, if it had a shape, what shape would it have?" etc
- "As you focus on that feeling where you feel it, on a scale of 0 – 10, how strong is it?"

We need this information because it will help us, and the client, to appreciate when the feeling reduces and by how much.

Talking the client through the process

You will explain that the client will be sitting with their eyes closed.

They will be noticing their normal gentle breath, and they will be imagining that they are 'breathing' into and out of different parts of their body as you guide them.

1. Start by getting them to close their eyes and ask them to focus their attention on that feeling in their body.

2. Ask them to imagine that they are breathing in and out of that feeling where they feel it. Let them do this for a few breaths.

3. Tell them to "try and hold on to that feeling", "hold on for as long as you can before it starts to disappear" [See Note]

4. Ask them to say to themselves, "I acknowledge this feeling and thank it for its contribution"

5. Now talk them through some breathing variations, described earlier. Focus your attention on their breathing and tell them in advance what they are to be doing: just before they start to breathe in, tell them to "breathe in through your crown" (for example), and before they exhale, tell them to "breathe out through the base of your spine". You don't need to tell them for every breath.

6. Your attention is on the client and you can see how they are breathing; you are looking at their face and their chest. You will notice when they take a deep sigh, for example, or if there is perhaps a welling up of emotion for a moment, or a deepening of their relaxation, or a tensing up even. This means that the energy of the emotion is altering. When this happens, use phrases like "that's it" or "just let that happen" [See Note]

7. Other useful suggestions that you could make would be: "and just start to notice those changes", "just allowing that feeling to move, ease, dissipate", "and just allow that feeling to soften, melt... that's it... just let that happen" etc

So you will go through three stages with them:

1. Have them breathe in/out of the feeling to begin with, and then move on to some variations.

2. Bring them back to breathing in/out of the feeling, and then try some more variations.

3. Finish by having them breathe in/out of the feeling, before asking them to open their eyes.

Ask them what changes they have noticed.

You are interested in knowing whether the feeling has changed its location in some way (it might have dissolved, spread and diluted itself, or even passed out of their body), you want to know of it feels different in some way (perhaps a change in shape or colour or texture) and you want to know how strong the feeling now is, on a scale of 0 – 10.

Repeat the breathing exercise again, and re-check.

If the feeling has reduced to zero, have the client "try and get the feeling back". Encourage them: "this is a familiar feeling, isn't it? You've had it for a long time… get it back"

They may not be able to do this, or if they do then the feeling will be less strong.

Repeat the breathing exercise until they can't get it back, or until it is at a sort of level that the client is happy with.

The idea here is that you are using their breathing to control and move their own energy to disrupt and fragment the energy of the unhelpful feeling, helping it to soften, loosen, disintegrate or dissolve.

Special language to use

Some of the phrases I have suggested might seem a little strange, but they are there for a reason. At the start of the technique I suggested these phrases:

- Try and hold on to that feeling
- Hold on for as long as you can before it starts to fade

Suggesting that someone 'try' something presupposes failure, and so telling someone to fail at holding onto the feeling is a useful thing to do; equally, the second suggestion presupposes that the feeling is going to fade.

Later on, as you notice changes in their breathing, or relaxation, or a deep sigh, or a moment of emotion, I suggested these phrases:

- That's it...
- Let that happen...
- That's good, just let that happen...

You don't know what's happening inside, but you know that the energy of the emotion is altering in some way and we want to encourage that.

You can usefully also make other suggestions, revolving around them noticing changes.

You might say, "that's it, just let that happen, just noticing all the things that are changing, as that feeling can start to soften, or ease, just dissolving and disintegrating with each breath you take… that's it… letting that feeling move and fragment, diluting and calming…and you can just start to notice that happen now…"

Working with a feeling on a number of occasions

A negative feeling will not always reduce to zero during one session and that's fine. Some feelings may need to be worked on over a number of occasions before they resolve.

Working with other feelings or beliefs that arise

Occasionally you might find that the feeling you are working on disappears, but when the client thinks of the event associated with that old feeling, a new negative feeling arises.

You can work on the new feeling until it is eliminated.

Occasionally you might find that there is another feeling or belief that is holding the client back, perhaps "I can't let this feeling go" or "I don't want to let this go" or "This can't resolve as quickly as this" (a belief that change can't happen so quickly).

If you phrase this as a feeling - "I feel like I can't let this go" – then you can work on that feeling, establishing where it is, what it's like, how strong it is, and reducing that to zero using the breathing technique, before returning to deal with what is left of the original negative feeling, no longer held back by that limiting belief/feeling.

Will this still work for non-Reiki people?

This method will work whether or not the client is attuned to Reiki.

If they are attuned to Reiki, then Reiki will click in and follow their breath and where their focus is, and enhance the process.

If they are not attuned to Reiki, they will be focusing and guiding their own chi, and your attention is on them and their feeling, you are following their breathing, and your Reiki will follow your focus and be channelled to them, rather like the 'Radiating Reiki' exercise that we teach on Second Degree.

Working with physical pain

One of my students has been using the breathing technique on some clients who have physical – rather than emotional – pain, to good effect.

How to use the breathing method with Reiki clients

I have to say that what I have been describing is quite an unusual thing for a Reiki person to do with a client. And clients are used to lying on a treatment couch, closing their eyes, and drifting off as you proceed with their treatment.

So here I suggest three different ways in which this method can be used with your Reiki clients.

Seated approach

When I have taught this method, I have had students sitting near each other, talking each other through the exercise and watching each other's breathing.

We can use this approach with a client too, formally dealing with an unhelpful emotion, separate from the Reiki treatment that takes place on the treatment table.

Client on the treatment table

This breathing method can be carried out with the client on a treatment table.

You can rest your hands on their shoulders throughout the process for a reassuring Reiki touch, you can talk them through the process, watching their breathing, watching their reactions and reacting to that with the things that you say to them as the emotion drains away.

If you like, you might actually rest your hands on or over the area of the body where they can feel the negative emotion, and focus the energy there.

While resting your hands on the shoulders, you would be directing the energy to that area using intent, of course.

Impromptu use, with an emotional release

It is also possible to use Reiki Emotional Integration when the client is starting to have an emotional release on the treatment table.

You can explain to them that you are now going to use a technique that will drain that strong emotion away for them.

1. Ask questions to establish where they have the feeling, what it's like and how strong it is.
2. Talk them through the breathing exercise and variations, using what suggestions seem appropriate.
3. Check to see how the feeling has changed.
4. Repeat the breathing exercise to reduce the feeling to a low level, or zero.
5. Have the client try and bring the feeling back, and deal with any remaining emotion as appropriate.

Combining the breathing method with the "three questions"

The next stage of our approach involves combining the three questions with this breathing method.

As you talk the client through the breathing exercises you will be channelling just the energy that they need in that moment, using the symbol and colour questions; for location, use the part of the body where the client says that they feel the feeling that they have.

So, having asked the client to locate and describe their feeling and calibrate the intensity of it, you explain the process and start them breathing in and out of their feeling/location.

As they are doing this, ask yourself the questions you need to ask to elicit just the energy that "they need in this moment" and start to direct this energy/symbol/colour on the location where they have the feeling; you can hover your hands near that area if you like.

You will be talking the client through the breathing exercise, making various suggestions, so you do not need to keep on reminding yourself of what the symbol and colour etc are – your intent is sufficient here.

And as the location of the feeling alters during the breathing sessions, reported to you when you ask for feedback, you

182

can alter where you are directing the energy for the next set of 'passes'.

An alternative set-up for the energy would be: "if the energy that they need to release this emotion had a shape…" etc

Providing a 'solution state' to your client

We can move the process just one stage further, once the client has reduced their negative emotion/state to a low level.

We can replace that emotion by whatever state/quality the client would like to experience instead.

So, for example, low self-esteem might be replaced by self-confidence, anxiety might be replaced by contentment.

Instead of eliminating a negative emotion and leaving them with a 'void', an absence of a negative thing, we can introduce a positive state.

Ask the client what they would like to feel instead of that feeling that they used to have.

The client just sits quietly and you ask the three questions, finding the symbol, colour and location that is best suited to this positive state.

Channel the energy using your hands, and radiating the energy out of your body, for as long as seems appropriate. You might choose to rest your hands on their shoulders at this stage.

A final thought about bespoke symbols

So, you have seen that you do not need to be attuned for a symbol for it to work for you and frame the energy in a particular way.

You have discovered that by asking yourself three questions you can elicit just the energy that you or your client needs in this moment, and you can frame the energy to work as a 'carrier' for various positive states or qualities.

You have learned a simple breathing method that you and your client can use to shift an unhelpful emotion or state, and you can enhance the effectiveness of this for your client by using various verbal suggestions and by channelling the energy that they need, as they go through the breathing exercise.

Finally, having helped reduce the strength of an unhelpful emotion to a low level, you can channel energy to provide the client – or yourself, remember - with a positive 'solution' state or emotion, replacing the old energy with a new, positive one.

Exploring the weird hypnotic language I was using

Modern hypnotherapy uses quite extensively a language form that derives from the work of Milton Erickson, an American and one of the most famous and revered Hypnotherapists.

He used language in an exquisite way to help his clients accept the 'suggestions' he made to them about how they might change their behaviour, thoughts, emotions for the better.

Before Erickson came along, Hypnotherapists gave people 'direct suggestions'. They tried to get clients into a very deep state of trance and then told them things, like, "you will feel calm when you stand up in front of a group of people" or "you will walk right past the sweets in the supermarket".

But people don't like to be told what to do, particularly when the instructions go against how things have been for them recently, and Erickson found a way to create useful verbal suggestions that slide 'under the radar', to be accepted more readily by his clients' subconscious minds.

Presuppositions

When we say to the client that they should "try" to hold on to that feeling, we are presupposing failure. The word "try" presupposes failure and we are suggesting that they are going to fail to hold onto the feeling.

We say, "hold onto that feeling for as long as you can before it starts to fade". This presupposes that the feeling is going to fade.

Artful vagueness

When we are talking a client through the breathing method and we notice that they sigh a deep sigh, or relax visibly, or tense up, we know that something is happening and we want to encourage that.

We can say, "just let that happen…". We don't know exactly what is happening but the client does and their unconscious minds can 'fill in the gaps'

We might say, "and you can notice those changes…". We don't know if there are changes going on, but that statement presupposes that there are changes and we leave it to the client's subconscious mind to interpret their experiences in terms of things changing, which is what we want.

Possibility

Notice that in the suggestion above, we said, "you can notice those changes…". We didn't say, "YOU WILL NOTICE THOSE CHANGES".

We were introducing a possibility, which is accepted by someone's unconscious mind a lot more readily, and we could have said, "you might notice those changes".

Words like can, could, may, might, all introduce useful suggestions as possibilities, which the unconscious mind accepts more readily and is more likely to act upon.

Using time

Another way of making a suggestion more 'slippery' and more acceptable to someone's unconscious mind is to say something like, "and you can start to notice those things that mean the feeling is dissolving now".

You're not saying that they will notice something, you are saying that they can and you're not even suggesting that they can feel something fully, just that they can start to notice something.

All these suggestions help to ease the process along, and work brilliantly with the energy work that you and your client are carrying out at the same time.

Experiencing & directing energy

Experiencing energy

I thought I would just spend a little while talking about the many ways in which Reiki can be experienced and can be controlled or directed by us.

Reiki is a very malleable and accommodating energy and does not require us to practise in a very narrow or well-defined way. There is no right way that you *have* to work with the energy. There is no *should*. There is no *must*.

Reiki moulds itself to very many ways of working and will even kick in and start flowing when we carry out other movement-based or healing or meditative practices. Reiki doesn't mind!

So, once a student has been on a Reiki course and has been initiated in some way, they are usually able to experience the flow of energy (they can usually 'feel something happening'), and, once 'connected', they will be working with energy, and experiencing energy, in different ways:

- When making movements
- Following your attention/focus
- Breathing
- Meditations
- Symbols
- Sounds
- Metaphor
- Bespoke symbolic systems

Movement

It's not uncommon for people who have been 'attuned' to Reiki to find that they become much more aware of the movement of energy when practicing Tai Chi or Qi Gong, or if they take up Tai Chi, for example, then they are aware of the flow of energy early on, much more than non-Reiki-attuned students.

Hand and arm movements turn up in other Reiki practices, for example in Kenyoku, in Reiju, in the Hara defining exercise and in the energy-ball self-empowerment method; hand and arm movements move energy and are an outer expression of an inner intent.

Following your attention or focus

"Where thought goes, energy flows" is a good dictum, and one way of experiencing this principle is when you allow your attention to rest or to dwell on a particular part of your body (or someone else's body) and the energy will flow there.

So, for example, when you practice the Usui Self-Treatment Meditation and allow your attention to come to rest on a particular part of your head, the energy flows there and many people can experience this as pressure or fizzing or tingling or a magnetic sensation.

You could do an exercise now: close your eyes and focus your attention on your third eye.

Feel yourself 'dwelling' there.

After a little while you should become aware of the energy focusing there, in whatever way you might experience it.

Now shift your attention to your throat area, or your heart area, and notice the energy focusing itself there.

Finally, bring your attention back to your third eye and experience the energy there.

When carrying out my "Reiki Inner Smile Meditation", when you allow your attention to come to rest on your inner organs, for example the lungs, the liver or the stomach, the energy focuses itself there, and people can become aware of the presence of Reiki building in those parts of the body.

Breathing

Something as simple as breathing involves the movement of energy, and one of the first things that a student does when they train with Reiki Evolution is to practice "Joshin Kokkyu ho", where they move energy to and from their Tanden, in time with their breath.

Here is a segment of an article that I wrote, entitled "Breath of earth and heaven", which you can find on the Reiki Evolution blog and in my book "Liberate Your Reiki!":

"Many people reading this article will be practising something called "Joshin Kokkyu Ho", an energy breathing method taught in the Usui Reiki Ryoho Gakkai, the Usui Memorial Society in Japan – part of a longer sequence of exercises referred to as "Hatsurei ho"

It was also used in Mikao Usui's original system, according to a group of Usui Sensei's surviving students who are in contact with one or two people in the West.

Joshin Kokkyu Ho translates as something like 'technique for purification of the spirit' or 'soul cleansing breathing method', and on its own 'Kokkyu Ho' means 'the way of breathing'.

When we use this method we are moving energy in time with our breath, into and out of our Tanden (Dantien in Chinese), it is a way of achieving balance, but there is more significance to this technique than simply moving energy through our bodies.

With each in-breath we are filling the body with ki. This ki is yin in nature, it is the breath of earth, of physicality and the power of separation.

By contrast the out-breath distributes ki throughout our bodies. This is yang in nature, it is the breath of heaven, of spirituality and the power of unification.

So from the moment that we practise Joshin Kokkyu Ho we are experiencing earth ki and heavenly ki. In fact, earth ki and heavenly ki are what we are: we are physical reality and we are spiritual essence.

In Taoist philosophy, Earth and Heaven – along with Humanity – are known as the "Three Powers". Humanity is in a pivotal position between the cosmic powers of heaven and the natural forces of earth, covered by heaven above and supported by earth below.

Qi Gong, the energy cultivation technique which is practised in Japan as 'kiko', allows us to work with these two energies and bring them into balance. Shinto practices also refer to these two basic energies, these two essential aspects of what we really are."

Meditations

Reiki is a meditative activity, and students use meditation to experience Reiki from the beginning of their training.

Joshin Kokkyu ho, Hatsurei ho and Mikao Usui's Self-treatment meditation are all ways of focusing and directing the energy through visualisation or intention (they are equivalent).

When meditating using Reiki, we are not 'flavouring' the energy in a particular way: we are allowing the energy to flow and to take whatever form it needs to take to benefit us.

Symbols

Reiki is endlessly malleable and by using some sort of visual representation or shape or 'graphic' we can frame the energy in a particular way.

CKR and SHK mould the energy in a particular way, by emphasising earth ki or heavenly ki, though HSZSN does not so much produce/elicit an energy so much as bring an experience of oneness.

We use symbol meditations, for example on Second Degree, as a self-healing practice.

Symbols from other traditions will mould or frame Reiki in a particular way, and for examples of this you might think of the Fire Dragon or the 'Tibetan' Master symbol, or channelled symbols, for example those that I use with my "Five Element Reiki" system.

Various new Reiki systems are based on different collections of systems, for example William Rand's "Karuna".

With or without an accompanying mantra, a shape or graphic or symbol will produce a particular energy signature or 'frequency'.

Earlier in this book, you were guided to experiment with the circle, square and triangle shapes and you meditated on and experienced their energies.

So you don't need to be attuned to a symbol (i.e. having the symbol inserted into you in some way during an attunement ritual) for it to mould the energy in a particular way.

Once you are connected to Reiki, in whatever way that was achieved, then any symbol will frame the energy for you.

And of course you do not need to take part in a ritual that involves the use of a symbol in order to be 'connected' to Reiki.

Sounds

There is something very special, very primal, about using sound to elicit energy: we are using vibrations to elicit 'vibrations', though you can also chant very effectively 'in your head' to elicit energy.

Reiki has its own set of ancient sounds in the form of the kotodama, Shinto mantras that were taught by Usui Sensei to more students than ever were taught symbols by him.

Many people find the Reiki kotodama to be something very special, powerful, bringing energy from within in a way that simply does not seem to happen when symbols are used.

In fact, many sounds can frame the energy in a particular way, producing a particular 'frequency' or energy signature.

Meditate on some new sounds

Various sounds are associated with the chakras, and it can be an interesting exercise to chant these sounds and feel the Reiki focusing itself on these energy centres.

Here is a guide to the sounds that correspond to each chakra:

Chakra	Corresponding sound
Root	UH as in 'huh'
Navel	OOO as in 'you'
Solar plexus	OH as in 'go'
Heart	AH as in 'star'
Throat	EYE as in 'eye'
Third eye	AY as in 'day'
Crown	EEE as in 'me'

Spend a little while chanting the sounds out loud, noticing any changes in your body as you do so, and then be still to experience the ongoing effects of the chanting.

Where do you experience the energy?
How does it make you feel?
What changes do you notice?

Metaphors

A metaphor isn't quite a symbol, but it is a way of representing different aspects of the energy in a visual fashion.

An example of this might be the 'Frequency scale meditation', taught on my Reiki Master Teacher course, where you bring into mind the idea that there is a sliding scale, with a little pointer or 'slider' that tracks up and down, representing different 'frequencies' of energy.

Low frequency energy is at the bottom of the scale; high frequencies are at the top, and other frequencies can be found in between in a sort of hierarchy.

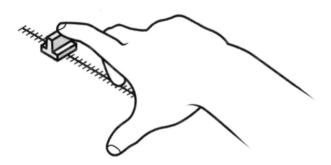

This metaphor is a way of working with intent, using the metaphor to represent, generate or elicit a particular 'frequency' of energy.

We can use different metaphors to get a handle on the energy and this is quite a useful way of representing something that might otherwise be fairly intangible.

The idea of 'frequencies' is another metaphor, of course, just a useful way of trying to describe or frame something intangible.

The energies may not actually be at different frequencies, but it can be useful to represent them to ourselves in that way.

Bespoke symbolic systems

If you have been working through this book in order, you will already have been exploring bespoke symbols and you will have experienced an energy based on 'just what I need in this moment', as well as an energy based on some desired characteristic, for example creativity.

You will have practised intuiting a graphical representation of some quality or state that you or your client would benefit from being immersed in.

You will not have been 'attuned' to these symbols, of course, nor do you need to be: they work for you perfectly well.

Directing energy

Following on from the above, I thought I would talk for a bit about the different ways in which we can control and direct the energy, with the proviso that I believe the best approach is always to work intuitively.

But I will talk more about that below.

So, here are the ways in which you can direct and control the energy:

The simplest approach

The simplest way to direct the energy, when treating someone, is to allow your attention to rest or to dwell on a particular part of their body.

When you treat someone, your attention is on them and you have set a particular intent: to channel energy for their benefit.

Energy flows.

When treating someone, for example while resting your hands on their shoulders, you can direct your attention towards another part of their body – for example their leg – and the energy will flow there.

While treating the temples you can imagine that there are additional hands cupped round the back of the recipient's head and hovering over the front of their face, and their head becomes engulfed by energy.

Here the 'construct', the visualizing or intending additional hands, is just a convenient way of focusing your attention, allowing your attention to dwell on the whole head.

The 'imaginary hands' method is optional since you can rest your attention 'direct' without using the intermediary of a metaphor like that.

Using symbols and sounds – why do we need to use them?

An important issue to deal with is why we might want to direct the energy in the first place using a symbol or a sound: if Reiki is drawn according to the recipient's need, giving them what they need on that occasion, and if the best approach is for us to get out of the way and allow it to happen, why would we want to wade in and use a symbol or a sound or a metaphor to frame the energy in a particular way?

Well, I believe that the best approach is to work in partnership with the energy, allowing your intuition/the energy/the recipient to guide you in terms of

1. Where you rest your hands
2. For how long you work in a particular position
3. What aspect of the energy, if any, you emphasise when working on someone

So whether you are using a particular hand position or staying in a particular hand position for a certain amount of time… or whether you are using a particular symbol, or a kotodama, or neither of those things… you are doing this because the energy guides you to.

The ideal, for me, is to work in partnership with the energy, following along with how it needs you to participate in the healing, doing the most appropriate and helpful thing that you can do to create the best sort of healing space for the recipient in that moment.

So you get your conscious mind out of the way, merge with the energy and the recipient, and allow to happen whatever then ensues.

So if it seems that a particular symbol, or sound, needs to be used – wants to be used – then you go with that. You are still 'out of the way', standing aside metaphorically to allow what needs to come through to come through, but you are following and working with the needs of the energy, emphasising what needs to be emphasised.

By 'directing' the energy intuitively you are not interfering with the flow: you are working with it.

So how might something come to mind?

Well, you might have a particular symbol come into your mind's eye, or become aware of a sound being chanted in your head, you might have a feeling or an impression that something needs to be focused on or emphasised.

Just go with that.

Beyond that, you are a neutral canvas, empty, with no expectations; you are merged with the energy and the recipient and allow it to happen.

If you like, perhaps not quite trusting your intuition yet, or just feeling your feet in this area, or because you like working this way, you might use a metaphor to check what seems to want to be used. For example, you might imagine four kotodama (in whatever way you might want to imagine them), say as four 'wands' resting on a table: look at the wands in your mind's eye and notice if any of them stand up, wanting to be used.

If none want to be used, don't use one.

Using symbols when you treat

The way that symbols are traditionally taught to be used in Western lineages is to draw out the symbol using your hands or finger(s), visualise the symbol being drawn out as you do that, and say the symbol's name to yourself usually silently) three times.

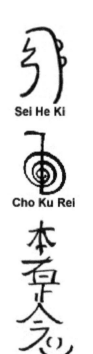

Sei He Ki

Cho Ku Rei

Hon Sha Ze Sho Nen

Dai Ko Myo

This is interesting because we know that people differ in terms of whether they work primarily in terms of visual images, sounds or kinaesthetic feelings.

Some people really can't visualise things, for example, whereas for others it is effortless. Drawing out a symbol, visualising it and saying its name touch all three 'representational system' bases and make the process one that will meet the needs of all practitioners.

Combining the three 'rep' systems together seems to work well for everyone.

My preferred way of using a symbol when treating is to hold the symbol up in the air above me, representing the 'source' of the energy.

You draw the symbol out in your mind (you can 'feel' it being drawn out or imagine that you are using your hands to do so, thus meeting the kinaesthetic need), see it being drawn out, and you say the symbol's name to yourself three times in your head.

Symbol sandwiches

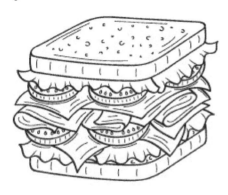

Mixing symbols together by putting one symbol on top of another really goes against the grain for me.

You have a perfectly-crafted image that elicits a particular energy signature or 'frequency' and then you take in and mix it up with other energy signatures, making a big old mess!

Symbol sandwiches are not a very Japanese way of doing things, where simplicity is the guiding principle, paring things down to the essentials.

If you imagine different symbols as being different pure colours of the rainbow, there are a couple of ways of looking at this:

1. Mixing together different rainbow colours of paint means you end up with grey-brown sludge in the end, and that's no use to anybody
2. Mixing together lots of frequencies of light means you just end up with white light, which is what you had in the first place before you started to introduce the symbols.

We use a symbol to emphasise an aspect of the energy; the power and potency comes through narrowing the focus of the energy, like a laser beam.

Mix with other aspects of the energy and you no longer have a laser-beam focus, just a confused, wide-angle coverage, something less than the sum of the parts.

Using novel symbols

Earlier I described an exercise where you meditated on three novel symbols and experienced their characteristic 'signatures', noticing how they affected you and where they seemed to focus themselves. We used the example of a circle, a triangle and a square.

You could actually use these symbols to treat someone if you liked, now that you know about them, using whichever symbol wanted to be used.

You don't need to be attuned to a symbol (i.e. having the symbol inserted into you in some way during an attunement ritual) for it to mould the energy in a particular way.

Once you are connected to Reiki, in whatever way that was achieved, then any symbol will frame the energy for you.

So if you wanted to use a symbol from another Reiki system, or try it out at least, for yourself and for people that you work on, you can, without having to be specifically 'attuned' to it.

Using sounds when you treat

Kotodama would usually be chanted silently in your head as you treat, unless you have a quite accommodating client who is happy for you to chant out loud above them!

Even though you are chanting in your head, you can do so with an awareness of deep vibration within you, and the kotodama energies usually arise powerfully and immediately from within, whereas, for many people, the energies of symbols seem to develop less quickly and seemingly from without.

Renewing the 'trigger' when you treat

There is the temptation sometimes to keep on drawing out a symbol in your mind's eye to make sure that you've still 'got' the energy.

This can be counterproductive and is a bit OCD!

By using a symbol you have set your intent in terms of what aspect of the energy you wish to emphasise, and the energy will flow in accordance with that intent.

You can then just merge with the energy and let it happen.

You don't need to keep on frantically re-drawing the symbol in your mind for fear of forgetting what you wanted. By all means draw the symbol again if you feel that you need to, but don't make endless re-drawing your default approach because it takes you away from the lovely stillness and mindfulness of a Reiki treatment.

Chanting a kotodama repeatedly is a different matter I think because chant is such a primal activity and because chant is often used as a way of entering a meditative state. You are not so much renewing something that you had completed - like drawing out a symbol again - as merging with an ongoing mantra, rather like TM, where you run a mantra continuously in your head.

Chanting in your head seems to not distract you from the meditation, but deepens it.

Chant the sound for as long as it seems to want to be chanted and then be still, empty and neutral, letting the energy flow.

Using a metaphor when treating

You could use a metaphor when treating someone, for example a 'frequency scale'.

Ideally you would use the metaphor as an intuitive device, so you notice where the slider wants to rest, and then focus on that 'frequency' of energy.: you use the scale to intuit the right energy for the client, and then use that scale to emphasise that frequency.

The metaphor is simply a form of 'hook' to focus your intent.

This approach may suit some people, not others, and I'm not suggesting that this becomes a regular part of your routine. It is a complication but will suit some people.

'Pure' intent

We don't have to use any sort of a trigger when we work with energy.

If we are familiar with a particular energy (through practising experiencing that energy in whatever way we might do that – using a symbol or a sound to elicit the energy, perhaps) then we can notice that a particular energy is coming through and we can emphasise that energy, by allowing our attention to dwell on the nature of that energy, or we might feel guided to use a particular 'feel' of energy that we elicit from within.